*Welcome to the **"Zero Point Weight Loss Cookbook: Satisfying and Nutritious Meals for Every Occasion."** If you're looking to transform your eating habits without sacrificing flavor or satisfaction, you've come to the right place. This cookbook is designed to support your weight loss journey by offering a wide array of delicious recipes that are not only nutritious but also carry a 0 point value, making it easier for you to stay on track.*

In a world where diet trends come and go, finding a sustainable and enjoyable way to eat healthily can be challenging. This cookbook simplifies the process by providing recipes that are both easy to prepare and packed with flavor. Whether you're a seasoned cook or just starting in the kitchen, these recipes are crafted to be approachable and rewarding.

Inside, you'll discover over 110 recipes that cater to every meal and occasion. From hearty breakfasts that kickstart your day to satisfying dinners that end it on a high note, we've got you covered. You'll also find snacks and desserts that will keep your cravings at bay without derailing your progress. Each recipe focuses on wholesome ingredients and balanced nutrition, ensuring you get the most out of every bite.

We understand that the journey to a healthier lifestyle is personal and unique. That's why this cookbook is more than just a collection of recipes; it's a tool to help you embrace a new way of eating that feels good and tastes even better. The zero point system allows you to enjoy a variety of foods while managing your weight effectively, offering the flexibility to create meals that suit your preferences and dietary needs.

As you explore the pages of this cookbook, you'll find tips and tricks to make meal preparation simpler and more enjoyable. We've included nutritional information for each recipe to help you make informed choices. Our goal is to empower you with the knowledge and inspiration to make lasting changes that benefit your health and well-being.

*So, let's get started on this delicious adventure! Embrace the flavors, enjoy the process, and celebrate the journey to a healthier, happier you. The **"Zero Point Weight Loss Cookbook"** is here to make your path to wellness both satisfying and nutritious, one delightful meal at a time.*

1. Grilled chicken breast

Ingredients:

- 4 boneless, skinless chicken breasts
- 2 tbsp olive oil
- 1 tsp salt
- 1 tsp black pepper
- 1 tsp garlic powder
- 1 tsp dried oregano

Instructions:

1. Preheat grill to medium·high heat.

2. Pat the chicken breasts dry with paper towels and place in a shallow dish. Drizzle with olive oil and sprinkle evenly with salt, pepper, garlic powder, and oregano. Rub the seasonings all over the chicken.

3. Grill the chicken for 5·7 minutes per side, or until the internal temperature reaches 165°F. The chicken should be cooked through and juices should run clear.

4. Transfer the grilled chicken breasts to a clean plate and let rest for 5 minutes before serving.

Serve the grilled chicken breasts as is, or slice and use in salads, sandwiches, or other recipes. Enjoy!

2. Baked fish (such as cod, tilapia, or salmon)

Ingredients:

• 4 (4•6 oz) fish fillets (cod, tilapia, or salmon)
• 1 tbsp olive oil
• 1 tsp lemon juice
• 1 tsp dried parsley
• 1/2 tsp garlic powder
• 1/4 tsp salt
• 1/4 tsp black pepper

Instructions:

1. Preheat oven to 400°F. Lightly grease a baking sheet or oven•safe dish.

2. Pat the fish fillets dry with paper towels and place them on the prepared baking sheet or dish.

3. In a small bowl, mix together the olive oil, lemon juice, parsley, garlic powder, salt, and pepper.

4. Brush or spoon the seasoning mixture evenly over the top of the fish fillets.

5. Bake for 12•15 minutes, or until the fish is opaque and flakes easily with a fork. Cooking time may vary depending on the thickness of the fillets.

6. Serve the baked fish immediately, garnished with extra lemon wedges if desired.

This baked fish recipe is a great 0 point weight loss meal when paired with steamed vegetables or a fresh salad. The simple seasoning allows the natural flavor of the fish to shine through. Enjoy!

3. Steamed shrimp

Ingredients:

- 1 lb raw shrimp, peeled and deveined
- 1 cup water
- 1 tbsp lemon juice
- 1 tsp garlic powder
- 1/2 tsp salt
- 1/4 tsp black pepper

Instructions:

1. Fill a steamer pot or large saucepan with 1 cup of water. Bring the water to a boil over high heat.

2. While the water is heating, place the shrimp in a steamer basket or colander that fits inside the pot.

3. In a small bowl, mix together the lemon juice, garlic powder, salt, and pepper.

4. Once the water is boiling, carefully place the steamer basket or colander with the shrimp over the boiling water. Cover and steam for 5•7 minutes, until the shrimp are opaque and cooked through.

5. Transfer the steamed shrimp to a serving bowl. Drizzle the lemon•garlic seasoning over the top and toss gently to coat.

6. Serve the steamed shrimp warm, with lemon wedges on the side if desired.

This steamed shrimp recipe is a fantastic 0 point weight loss meal. The simple seasoning allows the natural sweetness of the shrimp to shine. Pair it with a fresh salad or steamed vegetables for a complete and healthy meal.

4. Turkey breast slices

Ingredients:

• 1 lb turkey breast, sliced into 1/2•inch thick slices
• 1 tsp olive oil
• 1 tsp dried thyme
• 1/2 tsp garlic powder
• 1/4 tsp salt
• 1/4 tsp black pepper

Instructions:

1. Preheat your oven to 400°F. Line a baking sheet with parchment paper or a silicone baking mat.

2. In a small bowl, mix together the olive oil, thyme, garlic powder, salt, and pepper.

3. Place the turkey breast slices on the prepared baking sheet. Brush or drizzle the seasoning mixture evenly over the top of the turkey slices.

4. Bake for 12•15 minutes, flipping the slices halfway through, until the turkey is cooked through and reaches an internal temperature of 165°F.

5. Remove the baked turkey slices from the oven and let them rest for 5 minutes before serving.

This simple baked turkey breast recipe is a great 0 point weight loss meal. The turkey is lean protein and the seasoning adds lots of flavor without adding any extra calories or points.

Serve the turkey slices on their own, or use them in salads, wraps, or other dishes. They also make a great protein•packed snack.

5. Egg white omelette

Ingredients:

• 3 egg whites
• 1 tbsp water
• 1/4 tsp salt
• 1/8 tsp black pepper
• Cooking spray

Optional Fillings:
• Diced vegetables (such as spinach, tomatoes, onions, peppers)
• Lean protein (such as turkey, ham, or shredded chicken)
• Herbs (such as parsley, chives, or basil)
• Low•fat cheese (such as feta or shredded mozzarella)

Instructions:

1. Crack the egg whites into a small bowl and add the water, salt, and pepper. Whisk until well combined.

2. Spray a small non•stick skillet or omelet pan with cooking spray and heat over medium heat.

3. Pour the egg white mixture into the hot pan. As the eggs start to set around the edges, use a spatula to gently push the cooked edges towards the center, tilting the pan to allow the uncooked egg to flow to the edges.

4. Once the bottom is set but the top is still a bit wet, add your desired fillings to one half of the omelet.

5. Use the spatula to fold the unfilled half of the omelet over the filled half.

6. Cook for 1•2 minutes more, until the omelet is set.

7. Slide the folded omelet onto a plate and serve immediately.

This egg white omelet is a great 0 point weight loss meal. You can customize the fillings to your liking, just be mindful of the point values of any additional ingredients. Enjoy!

6. Plain Greek yogurt

Ingredients:

Nutrition:
• 1 cup of plain, non•fat Greek yogurt contains:
• 100 calories
• 0g fat
• 18g protein
• 6g carbs
• 0g added sugar

Benefits for Weight Loss:
• High in protein • the protein helps keep you feeling full and satisfied, which can aid in weight loss.

• Low in calories and carbs • Greek yogurt is very low in calories and has minimal carbs, making it a great low•calorie, low•carb option.

• 0 points on many weight loss programs • plain Greek yogurt is typically a 0 point food on programs like Weight Watchers.

• Versatile • you can use plain Greek yogurt in sweet or savory dishes, as a dip, in smoothies, and more.

Tips for Enjoying:

• Choose plain, non•fat or low•fat Greek yogurt to keep it 0 points.

• Avoid flavored Greek yogurts, as they often contain added sugars.

• Top with fresh fruit, nuts, cinnamon, or a small drizzle of honey for flavor.

• Use it in recipes in place of sour cream, mayo, or cream cheese to save calories.

Plain Greek yogurt is an excellent 0 point weight loss food that provides protein, calcium, and other nutrients. It's a versatile and satisfying option to incorporate into a healthy diet.

7. Cottage cheese

Ingredients:

• 1 cup of low•fat cottage cheese contains:
• 163 calories
• 2.3g fat
• 28g protein
• 6g carbs
• 0g added sugar

Benefits for Weight Loss:
• High in protein • the protein in cottage cheese helps keep you feeling full and satisfied, which can aid in weight loss.

• Low in calories and fat • low•fat cottage cheese is very low in calories and fat, making it a great low•calorie option.

• 0 points on many weight loss programs • cottage cheese is typically a 0 point food on programs like Weight Watchers.

• Versatile • you can enjoy cottage cheese on its own or use it in sweet and savory dishes.

Tips for Enjoying:

• Choose low•fat or non•fat cottage cheese to keep it 0 points.

• Avoid cottage cheese with added sugars or flavorings, as those will increase the calorie and point count.

• Top with fresh fruit, nuts, cinnamon, or a small drizzle of honey for flavor.

• Use it in recipes in place of sour cream, mayo, or ricotta cheese to save calories.

Cottage cheese is an excellent 0 point weight loss food that provides protein, calcium, and other important nutrients. It's a versatile and satisfying option to incorporate into a healthy diet.

8. Mixed green salad (with zero•point dressing)

Ingredients:

• 2 cups mixed greens (such as spinach, kale, romaine, etc.)
• Assorted vegetables (such as tomatoes, cucumbers, bell peppers, onions, etc.)
• Zero•point dressing (such as balsamic vinegar, lemon juice, or a simple vinaigrette)

Instructions:

1. Wash and chop the mixed greens and any desired vegetables. Place them in a large salad bowl.

2. For the dressing, choose a zero•point option such as:
• Balsamic vinegar
• Lemon juice
• Red wine vinegar
• Apple cider vinegar
• Dijon mustard mixed with a small amount of olive oil

3. Drizzle the zero•point dressing over the salad and toss gently to coat.

Benefits for Weight Loss:

• Greens and vegetables are very low in calories and high in fiber, which helps keep you feeling full.

• Zero•point dressings add flavor without adding any calories or points.

• This salad makes for a satisfying, nutrient•dense meal that fits perfectly into a 0 point weight loss plan.

Tips:
• Avoid high•calorie, high•point dressings like ranch, creamy Italian, or thousand island.

• Add lean protein like grilled chicken, shrimp, or hard•boiled eggs to make it more filling.

• Top with a sprinkle of nuts or seeds for healthy fats and crunch.

A mixed green salad with a zero•point dressing is an excellent 0 point weight loss meal. It's filling, nutritious, and can be customized to your taste preferences.

9. Cucumber slices

Ingredients:

• 1 cup of sliced cucumber contains:
• 16 calories
• 0g fat
• 1g protein
• 4g carbs
• 0g added sugar

Benefits for Weight Loss:
• Very low in calories • cucumbers are one of the most low•calorie vegetables you can eat.

• High in water content • cucumbers are made up of about 95% water, which helps keep you hydrated and feeling full.

• 0 points on many weight loss programs • cucumbers are typically a 0 point food on programs like Weight Watchers.

• Versatile • you can enjoy cucumber slices on their own as a snack or incorporate them into salads, sandwiches, and more.

Tips for Enjoying:

• Choose fresh, crisp cucumbers and slice them into rounds or sticks.

• For extra flavor, you can sprinkle the cucumber slices with a bit of lemon juice, vinegar, salt, and pepper.

• Pair cucumber slices with a 0 point dip like plain Greek yogurt or hummus for a satisfying snack.

• Add cucumber slices to salads, wraps, or sandwiches for a refreshing crunch.

Cucumber slices are an excellent 0 point weight loss food that provide hydration, fiber, and very few calories. They're a great option to have on hand for healthy snacking or to incorporate into your meals.

10. Bell pepper strips

Ingredients:

• 1 cup of sliced bell peppers contains:
• 52 calories
• 0g fat
• 2g protein
• 12g carbs
• 0g added sugar

Benefits for Weight Loss:
• Very low in calories • bell peppers are one of the most low•calorie vegetables you can eat.

• High in fiber and water content • bell peppers are high in fiber and made up of about 92% water, which helps keep you feeling full.

• 0 points on many weight loss programs • bell peppers are typically a 0 point food on programs like Weight Watchers.

• Nutrient•dense • bell peppers are packed with vitamins, minerals, and antioxidants.

• Versatile • you can enjoy bell pepper strips on their own as a snack or incorporate them into salads, stir•fries, and more.

Tips for Enjoying:

• Choose a variety of colored bell peppers (red, yellow, orange, green) for maximum nutrition.

• Slice the bell peppers into long, thin strips for easy snacking.

• For extra flavor, you can sprinkle the bell pepper strips with a bit of lemon juice, vinegar, salt, and pepper.

• Pair bell pepper strips with a 0 point dip like hummus or tzatziki for a satisfying snack.

• Add bell pepper strips to salads, wraps, or stir•fries for a crunchy, flavorful addition.

Bell pepper strips are an excellent 0 point weight loss food that provide fiber, vitamins, and very few calories. They're a great option to have on hand for healthy snacking or to incorporate into your meals.

11. Sugar snap peas

Ingredients:

- 1 lb sugar snap peas, trimmed
- 1 tbsp water
- 1/4 tsp salt
- 1/8 tsp black pepper

Instructions:

1. Bring a medium saucepan filled with 1 inch of water to a boil over high heat.

2. Add the trimmed sugar snap peas to a steamer basket or colander that fits inside the saucepan.

3. Carefully place the steamer basket or colander with the peas over the boiling water. Cover and steam for 3•5 minutes, until the peas are tender•crisp.

4. Transfer the steamed sugar snap peas to a serving bowl. Drizzle with the 1 tbsp of water and season with the salt and black pepper. Toss gently to coat.

5. Serve the steamed sugar snap peas warm or at room temperature.

Benefits of Sugar Snap Peas for Weight Loss:

- Very low in calories • 1 cup of sugar snap peas has only 26 calories.

- High in fiber • the fiber in sugar snap peas helps keep you feeling full.

- 0 points on many weight loss programs • sugar snap peas are typically a 0 point food.

- Nutrient•dense • sugar snap peas are a good source of vitamins A, C, and K.

This simple steamed sugar snap pea recipe is a great 0 point weight loss snack or side dish. You can also enjoy them raw with a 0 point dip like hummus or tzatziki. Enjoy!

12. Baby carrots

Ingredients:

• 1 lb baby carrots, peeled and trimmed
• 1 tsp olive oil
• 1/4 tsp salt
• 1/8 tsp black pepper

Instructions:

1. Preheat your oven to 400°F. Line a baking sheet with parchment paper or a silicone baking mat.

2. Place the baby carrots on the prepared baking sheet. Drizzle with the olive oil and sprinkle with the salt and pepper. Toss to coat the carrots evenly.

3. Roast the baby carrots for 15•20 minutes, stirring halfway, until they are tender and lightly browned.

4. Remove the roasted baby carrots from the oven and serve warm.

Benefits of Baby Carrots for Weight Loss:

• Very low in calories • 1 cup of baby carrots has only 50 calories.

• High in fiber and water content – the fiber and water help keep you feeling full.

• 0 points on many weight loss programs – baby carrots are typically a 0 point food.

• Nutrient•dense – baby carrots are an excellent source of vitamins A, C, and K.

This roasted baby carrot recipe is a great 0 point weight loss snack or side dish. You can also enjoy baby carrots raw with a 0 point dip like hummus or tzatziki. The natural sweetness of the carrots makes them a satisfying and healthy option.

13. Celery sticks

Ingredients:

• 1 bunch of celery, washed and cut into 4•inch sticks

Optional Toppings/Dips:
• 2 tbsp natural peanut butter (0 points)
• 2 tbsp hummus (0 points)
• 2 tbsp plain Greek yogurt (0 points)
• Lemon juice, salt, and pepper

Instructions:

1. Wash the celery and cut the stalks into 4•inch sticks.

2. Arrange the celery sticks on a plate or in a container.

3. If desired, serve the celery sticks with a 0 point dip or topping such as:
• Natural peanut butter
• Hummus
• Plain Greek yogurt mixed with a squeeze of lemon juice, salt, and pepper

Benefits of Celery Sticks for Weight Loss:

• Extremely low in calories • 1 cup of celery sticks has only 16 calories.

• High in fiber and water content • the fiber and water help keep you feeling full.

• 0 points on many weight loss programs • celery sticks are typically a 0 point food.

• Crunchy and satisfying • the crisp texture makes celery sticks a great snack.

• Nutrient•dense • celery is a good source of vitamins, minerals, and antioxidants.

Celery sticks are a fantastic 0 point weight loss food that you can enjoy on their own or with a healthy, 0 point dip or topping. They make for a refreshing, crunchy, and satisfying snack.

14. Radishes

Ingredients:

• 1 lb radishes, trimmed and halved or quartered if large
• 1 tsp olive oil
• 1/4 tsp salt
• 1/8 tsp black pepper

Instructions:

1. Preheat your oven to 400°F. Line a baking sheet with parchment paper.

2. In a medium bowl, toss the trimmed and halved/quartered radishes with the olive oil, salt, and pepper until evenly coated.

3. Spread the seasoned radishes in a single layer on the prepared baking sheet.

4. Roast the radishes for 15•20 minutes, stirring halfway, until they are tender and lightly browned.

5. Remove the roasted radishes from the oven and serve warm.

Benefits of Radishes for Weight Loss:

• Very low in calories • 1 cup of raw radishes has only 19 calories.

• High in fiber • the fiber in radishes helps keep you feeling full.

• 0 points on many weight loss programs • radishes are typically a 0 point food.

• Crunchy and refreshing • the crisp texture makes radishes a great snack.

• Nutrient•dense • radishes are a good source of vitamins, minerals, and antioxidants.

Roasted radishes are a delicious 0 point weight loss food. You can also enjoy raw radish slices or rounds with a 0 point dip like hummus or tzatziki. Radishes make a great crunchy, low•calorie addition to salads, sandwiches, and more.

15. Cherry tomatoes

Ingredients:

• 1 pint cherry tomatoes, halved
• 1 tsp olive oil
• 1/4 tsp salt
• 1/8 tsp black pepper

Instructions:

1. Preheat your oven to 400°F. Line a baking sheet with parchment paper.

2. In a medium bowl, gently toss the halved cherry tomatoes with the olive oil, salt, and pepper until evenly coated.

3. Spread the seasoned cherry tomatoes in a single layer on the prepared baking sheet.

4. Bake for 12•15 minutes, until the tomatoes are softened and starting to burst.

5. Remove the baked cherry tomatoes from the oven and serve warm or at room temperature.

Benefits of Cherry Tomatoes for Weight Loss:

• Very low in calories • 1 cup of cherry tomatoes has only 27 calories.

• High in fiber and water content • the fiber and water help keep you feeling full.

• 0 points on many weight loss programs • cherry tomatoes are typically a 0 point food.

• Nutrient•dense • cherry tomatoes are a good source of vitamins, minerals, and antioxidants.

• Versatile • you can enjoy cherry tomatoes raw, roasted, or in a variety of dishes.

Baked cherry tomatoes make a delicious 0 point weight loss snack or side dish. You can also enjoy them raw with a 0 point dip like hummus or tzatziki. Cherry tomatoes are a great way to add flavor, texture, and nutrition to your meals.

16. Steamed broccoli

Ingredients:

• 1 lb broccoli florets
• 1 tbsp water
• 1/4 tsp salt
• 1/8 tsp black pepper

Instructions:

1. Fill a medium saucepan with about 1 inch of water and bring it to a boil over high heat.

2. Place the broccoli florets in a steamer basket or colander that fits inside the saucepan.

3. Carefully lower the steamer basket or colander into the boiling water. Cover and steam the broccoli for 5•7 minutes, until it is tender•crisp.

4. Transfer the steamed broccoli to a serving bowl. Drizzle with the 1 tbsp of water and season with the salt and black pepper. Toss gently to coat.

5. Serve the steamed broccoli warm.

Benefits of Steamed Broccoli for 0 Point Weight Loss:

• Extremely low in calories • 1 cup of steamed broccoli has only 55 calories.

• High in fiber • the fiber in broccoli helps keep you feeling full.

• 0 points on many weight loss programs • steamed broccoli is typically a 0 point food.

• Nutrient•dense • broccoli is packed with vitamins, minerals, and antioxidants.

• Versatile • you can enjoy steamed broccoli on its own or incorporate it into a variety of dishes.

This simple steamed broccoli recipe is a fantastic 0 point weight loss meal. You can enjoy it as a side dish or incorporate it into a larger meal. The possibilities are endless!

17. Steamed cauliflower

Ingredients:

• 1 lb cauliflower florets
• 1 tbsp water
• 1/4 tsp salt
• 1/8 tsp black pepper

Instructions:

1. Fill a medium saucepan with about 1 inch of water and bring it to a boil over high heat.

2. Place the cauliflower florets in a steamer basket or colander that fits inside the saucepan.

3. Carefully lower the steamer basket or colander into the boiling water. Cover and steam the cauliflower for 5•7 minutes, until it is tender•crisp.

4. Transfer the steamed cauliflower to a serving bowl. Drizzle with the 1 tbsp of water and season with the salt and black pepper. Toss gently to coat.

5. Serve the steamed cauliflower warm.

Benefits of Steamed Cauliflower for 0 Point Weight Loss:

• Extremely low in calories • 1 cup of steamed cauliflower has only 29 calories.

• High in fiber • the fiber in cauliflower helps keep you feeling full.

• 0 points on many weight loss programs • steamed cauliflower is typically a 0 point food.

• Nutrient•dense • cauliflower is packed with vitamins, minerals, and antioxidants.

• Versatile • you can enjoy steamed cauliflower on its own or incorporate it into a variety of dishes.

This simple steamed cauliflower recipe is a fantastic 0 point weight loss meal. You can enjoy it as a side dish or incorporate it into a larger meal. The possibilities are endless!

18. Asparagus spears

Ingredients:

• 1 lb asparagus spears, trimmed
• 1 tsp olive oil
• 1/4 tsp salt
• 1/8 tsp black pepper

Instructions:

1. Preheat your oven to 400°F. Line a baking sheet with parchment paper.

2. In a medium bowl, toss the trimmed asparagus spears with the olive oil, salt, and pepper until evenly coated.

3. Spread the seasoned asparagus in a single layer on the prepared baking sheet.

4. Roast the asparagus for 10•12 minutes, flipping halfway, until it is tender•crisp.

5. Remove the roasted asparagus from the oven and serve warm.

Benefits of Asparagus for 0 Point Weight Loss:

• Very low in calories • 1 cup of asparagus has only 40 calories.

• High in fiber • the fiber in asparagus helps keep you feeling full.

• 0 points on many weight loss programs • asparagus is typically a 0 point food.

• Nutrient•dense • asparagus is packed with vitamins, minerals, and antioxidants.

• Versatile • you can enjoy asparagus roasted, steamed, or incorporated into a variety of dishes.

This simple roasted asparagus recipe is a fantastic 0 point weight loss meal. You can also enjoy asparagus steamed with a squeeze of lemon juice or as part of a larger vegetable•based dish.

19. Zucchini noodles (zoodles)

Ingredients:

• 2 medium zucchinis, spiralized or julienned into noodle shapes
• 1 tsp olive oil
• 1/4 tsp salt
• 1/8 tsp black pepper

Optional Toppings:
• Marinara sauce
• Pesto
• Grilled chicken or shrimp
• Parmesan cheese

Instructions:

1. Use a spiralizer, julienne peeler, or vegetable peeler to cut the zucchinis into long, thin noodle shapes.

2. In a large skillet, heat the olive oil over medium heat. Add the zucchini noodles and season with the salt and pepper.

3. Cook the zucchini noodles for 3•5 minutes, stirring frequently, until they are tender•crisp.

4. Transfer the zucchini noodles to a serving bowl or plate. Top with your desired sauce, protein, or other toppings.

Benefits of Zucchini Noodles for 0 Point Weight Loss:

• Very low in calories • 1 cup of zucchini noodles has only 19 calories.

• High in fiber and water content • the fiber and water help keep you feeling full.

• 0 points on many weight loss programs • zucchini noodles are typically a 0 point food.

• Nutrient•dense • zucchini is a good source of vitamins, minerals, and antioxidants.

• Versatile • you can use zucchini noodles in place of pasta in a variety of dishes.

Zucchini noodles are a fantastic 0 point weight loss alternative to traditional pasta. They're easy to prepare and can be enjoyed with a variety of sauces and toppings for a satisfying and healthy meal.

20. Spaghetti squash

Ingredients:

• 1 medium spaghetti squash, halved lengthwise and seeds removed
• 1 tsp olive oil
• 1/4 tsp salt
• 1/8 tsp black pepper

Instructions:

1. Preheat your oven to 400°F. Line a baking sheet with parchment paper.

2. Place the spaghetti squash halves cut•side up on the prepared baking sheet. Drizzle the olive oil over the squash and sprinkle with the salt and pepper.

3. Roast the spaghetti squash for 40•50 minutes, until it is tender and can be easily shredded with a fork.

4. Remove the roasted spaghetti squash from the oven and let it cool slightly. Use a fork to shred the flesh into long, spaghetti•like strands.

5. Transfer the spaghetti squash strands to a serving bowl. You can top them with your desired 0 point sauces, proteins, or vegetables.

Benefits of Spaghetti Squash for 0 Point Weight Loss:

• Very low in calories • 1 cup of cooked spaghetti squash has only 42 calories.

• High in fiber • the fiber in spaghetti squash helps keep you feeling full.

• 0 points on many weight loss programs • spaghetti squash is typically a 0 point food.

• Nutrient•dense • spaghetti squash is a good source of vitamins, minerals, and antioxidants.

• Versatile • you can use spaghetti squash in place of pasta in a variety of dishes.

Roasted spaghetti squash is a fantastic 0 point weight loss alternative to traditional pasta. It's easy to prepare and can be enjoyed with a variety of sauces and toppings for a satisfying and healthy meal.

21. Lettuce wraps (using lean protein and veggies)

Ingredients:

• 1 lb lean ground turkey or chicken
• 1 tbsp low•sodium soy sauce or tamari
• 1 tsp sesame oil
• 1 tsp grated ginger
• 1 garlic clove, minced
• 1/4 tsp red pepper flakes (optional)
• 1 cup shredded carrots
• 1 cup thinly sliced cucumber
• 1/2 cup thinly sliced red bell pepper
• 12•16 large lettuce leaves (such as romaine, bibb, or butter lettuce)

Instructions:

1. In a large skillet over medium•high heat, cook the ground turkey or chicken, breaking it up as it cooks, until no longer pink, about 5•7 minutes.

2. Drain any excess fat from the pan, then stir in the soy sauce, sesame oil, ginger, garlic, and red pepper flakes (if using). Cook for 1•2 minutes more.

3. Remove the pan from heat and stir in the shredded carrots, sliced cucumber, and bell pepper.

4. To assemble the lettuce wraps, place a couple tablespoons of the turkey/veggie mixture into the center of a lettuce leaf. Fold the sides of the lettuce over the filling and enjoy.

Benefits of Lettuce Wraps for 0 Point Weight Loss:

• Lettuce leaves are very low in calories and 0 points.

• Lean protein like turkey or chicken provides filling, satisfying nutrition.

• Vegetables add fiber, vitamins, and minerals.

• You can customize the fillings to your taste preferences.

• Lettuce wraps are a great way to enjoy a satisfying meal without the extra calories and points from bread or tortillas.

This lettuce wrap recipe is a fantastic 0 point weight loss meal. Feel free to experiment with different protein and veggie combinations to keep things interesting. Enjoy!

22. Salsa (fresh or jarred)

Ingredients:

• 1/2 cup of fresh or jarred salsa typically contains:
• 25•50 calories
• 0g fat
• 1•2g protein
• 5•10g carbs
• 0g added sugar

Benefits for Weight Loss:
• Very low in calories • salsa is an extremely low•calorie condiment.

• High in fiber and water content • the vegetables in salsa provide fiber and hydration.

• 0 points on many weight loss programs • salsa is typically a 0 point food.

• Flavorful • salsa can add a lot of flavor to dishes without adding many calories.

• Versatile • you can enjoy salsa with a variety of 0 point foods like vegetables, eggs, or lean proteins.

Tips for Enjoying Salsa:

• Choose fresh or jarred salsas without added sugars or oils.

• Use salsa as a dip for raw veggies like carrots, celery, or bell pepper strips.

• Top grilled or baked chicken, fish, or tofu with salsa.

• Mix salsa into scrambled eggs or omelets.

• Use salsa as a topping for baked potatoes or spaghetti squash.

Salsa, whether fresh or jarred, is an excellent 0 point weight loss food that can add flavor and nutrition to your meals and snacks. It's a great way to enjoy bold, zesty flavors without the extra calories.

23. Bean sprouts

Ingredients:

- 1 cup of raw bean sprouts contains:
- 31 calories
- 0g fat
- 3g protein
- 6g carbs
- 0g added sugar

Benefits for Weight Loss:

- Very low in calories • bean sprouts are one of the most low•calorie vegetables.

- High in fiber and water content • the fiber and water help keep you feeling full.

- 0 points on many weight loss programs • bean sprouts are typically a 0 point food.

- Nutrient•dense • bean sprouts are a good source of vitamins, minerals, and antioxidants.

- Versatile • you can enjoy bean sprouts raw, cooked, or incorporated into a variety of dishes.

Tips for Enjoying Bean Sprouts:

- Rinse bean sprouts thoroughly before using to remove any dirt or debris.

- Enjoy bean sprouts raw in salads, wraps, or as a crunchy snack.

- Sauté or stir•fry bean sprouts with other vegetables and lean proteins.

- Add bean sprouts to soups, stir•fries, or noodle dishes for extra crunch and nutrition.

- Season bean sprouts with a bit of low•sodium soy sauce, rice vinegar, or lemon juice.

Bean sprouts are a fantastic 0 point weight loss food that can be enjoyed in a variety of ways. Their crunchy texture and mild flavor make them a versatile addition to many healthy meals and snacks.

24. Kale chips

Ingredients:

• 1 bunch of kale, washed and torn into bite•sized pieces
• 1 tsp olive oil
• 1/4 tsp salt

Instructions:

1. Preheat your oven to 350°F. Line a baking sheet with parchment paper.

2. In a large bowl, toss the kale pieces with the olive oil and salt until the kale is evenly coated.

3. Spread the kale in a single layer on the prepared baking sheet, making sure the pieces are not overlapping.

4. Bake for 12•15 minutes, flipping the kale halfway, until the kale is crispy and lightly browned.

5. Remove the kale chips from the oven and let them cool slightly before serving.

Benefits of Kale Chips for Weight Loss:

• Extremely low in calories • 1 cup of kale chips has only about 35 calories.

• High in fiber • the fiber in kale helps keep you feeling full.

• 0 points on many weight loss programs • kale chips are typically a 0 point food.

• Nutrient•dense • kale is packed with vitamins, minerals, and antioxidants.

• Satisfying crunch • the crispy texture of kale chips makes them a great cruchy snack.

Kale chips are a fantastic 0 point weight loss snack. They satisfy the craving for something crunchy and salty, without the extra calories and points. Feel free to experiment with different seasonings as well.

25. Roasted Brussels sprouts

Ingredients:

- 1 lb Brussels sprouts, trimmed and halved
- 1 tsp olive oil
- 1/4 tsp salt
- 1/8 tsp black pepper

Instructions:

1. Preheat your oven to 400°F. Line a baking sheet with parchment paper.

2. In a medium bowl, toss the trimmed and halved Brussels sprouts with the olive oil, salt, and pepper until evenly coated.

3. Spread the seasoned Brussels sprouts in a single layer on the prepared baking sheet.

4. Roast the Brussels sprouts for 18•22 minutes, stirring halfway, until they are tender and lightly browned.

5. Remove the roasted Brussels sprouts from the oven and serve warm.

Benefits of Roasted Brussels Sprouts for Weight Loss:

- Very low in calories • 1 cup of roasted Brussels sprouts has only 56 calories.

- High in fiber • the fiber in Brussels sprouts helps keep you feeling full.

- 0 points on many weight loss programs • Brussels sprouts are typically a 0 point food.

- Nutrient•dense • Brussels sprouts are packed with vitamins, minerals, and antioxidants.

- Versatile • you can enjoy roasted Brussels sprouts on their own or incorporate them into a variety of dishes.

This simple roasted Brussels sprouts recipe is a fantastic 0 point weight loss side dish or snack. The roasting brings out the natural sweetness of the sprouts, making them a delicious and nutritious option.

26. Roasted sweet potatoes (in moderation)

Ingredients:

• 2 medium sweet potatoes, peeled and cut into 1•inch cubes
• 1 tsp olive oil
• 1/4 tsp salt
• 1/8 tsp black pepper

Instructions:

1. Preheat your oven to 400°F. Line a baking sheet with parchment paper.

2. In a medium bowl, toss the cubed sweet potatoes with the olive oil, salt, and pepper until evenly coated.

3. Spread the seasoned sweet potato cubes in a single layer on the prepared baking sheet.

4. Roast the sweet potatoes for 20•25 minutes, flipping halfway, until they are tender and lightly browned.

5. Remove the roasted sweet potatoes from the oven and serve warm.

Benefits of Roasted Sweet Potatoes for Weight Loss:

• Moderate in calories • 1 cup of roasted sweet potatoes has about 103 calories.

• High in fiber and nutrients • sweet potatoes are a good source of fiber, vitamins, and minerals.

• Can be enjoyed in moderation on many weight loss programs • sweet potatoes are often a limited point food.

• Satisfying and versatile • roasted sweet potatoes make a great side dish or addition to meals.

While sweet potatoes are nutritious, they do contain more carbohydrates and calories than some other vegetables. It's important to enjoy them in moderation as part of a balanced 0 point weight loss plan. Stick to a 1/2 to 1 cup serving size.

27. Air•popped popcorn

Ingredients:

• 1/2 cup popcorn kernels

Instructions:

1. In an air popper machine, add the 1/2 cup of popcorn kernels.

2. Turn on the air popper and let it run until the popping slows to 2•3 seconds between pops.

3. Once the popping has finished, carefully remove the popped popcorn from the air popper's bowl.

4. Transfer the air•popped popcorn to a large bowl.

That's it! The air popper will do all the work of popping the kernels into light, fluffy popcorn.

Tips:
• Use high•quality popcorn kernels for best results.
• You can season the popcorn with a variety of toppings, such as:
  • Salt
  • Melted butter
  • Grated parmesan cheese
  • Garlic powder
  • Cajun seasoning
  • Nutritional yeast
• Store any leftover popcorn in an airtight container at room temperature for up to 3 days.

Air•popped popcorn is a healthy, low•calorie snack option. Enjoy it plain or with your favorite seasonings!

28. Edamame (plain, steamed)

Ingredients:

• 1 lb fresh edamame in the pod
• 1•2 tbsp coarse sea salt or kosher salt

Instructions:

1. Bring a large pot of water to a boil over high heat.

2. Add the edamame pods to the boiling water. Cover the pot with a lid and let the edamame steam for 5•7 minutes, until bright green and tender.

3. Drain the edamame in a colander and transfer to a serving bowl.

4. Sprinkle the coarse salt over the hot edamame pods. The salt will stick to the pods.

5. Serve the steamed edamame warm, with the salt. Provide small bowls for discarding the empty pods.

Tips:

• Look for fresh, bright green edamame pods. Avoid any that are yellowed or shriveled.

• You can adjust the cooking time based on your desired level of tenderness. 5 minutes will result in a firmer texture, while 7 minutes will be more soft and tender.

• For extra flavor, you can also toss the steamed edamame with a bit of soy sauce, sesame oil, or lemon juice.

• Edamame is a great high•protein, fiber•rich snack or appetizer. Enjoy!

29. Sugar•free gelatin

Ingredients:

• 1 (0.25 oz) packet of unflavored gelatin powder
• 1 cup cold water
• 1 cup boiling water
• 1 (3 oz) package of sugar•free gelatin mix (any flavor)

Instructions:

1. In a medium bowl, sprinkle the unflavored gelatin powder over the 1 cup of cold water. Let it sit for 5 minutes to bloom.

2. Add the 1 cup of boiling water to the bloomed gelatin and stir until the gelatin is completely dissolved, about 2•3 minutes.

3. Add the 3 oz package of sugar•free gelatin mix and stir until fully dissolved.

4. Pour the gelatin mixture into a lightly oiled 8x8 inch baking dish or individual ramekins.

5. Refrigerate the gelatin for at least 4 hours, or until completely set.

6. Once set, you can unmold the gelatin and serve as desired. Top with fresh fruit, whipped cream, or enjoy it plain.

Tips:
• Use any flavor of sugar•free gelatin mix that you prefer.

• For a firmer set, you can use 1 1/4 cups of boiling water instead of 1 cup.

• Experiment with adding fresh fruit, nuts, or other mix•ins to the gelatin.

• Store any leftover sugar•free gelatin covered in the refrigerator for up to 5 days.

This sugar•free gelatin is a great low•calorie, low•carb dessert option. Enjoy!

30. Pickles

Ingredients:

• 3 lbs cucumbers, sliced or cut into spears
• 1 cup white vinegar
• 1 cup water
• 2 tbsp salt
• 1 tbsp sugar
• 2 tsp dill seeds
• 2 garlic cloves, peeled and halved
• 1 tsp black peppercorns

Instructions:

1. Wash the cucumbers and slice or cut them into spears, depending on your preference.

2. In a large bowl, combine the vinegar, water, salt, and sugar. Stir until the salt and sugar have dissolved.

3. Add the sliced or speared cucumbers, dill seeds, garlic, and peppercorns to the vinegar mixture. Stir to combine.

4. Transfer the pickles to a clean, sterilized jar or container with a tight•fitting lid.

5. Refrigerate the pickles for at least 24 hours before serving. The longer they sit, the more flavorful they will become.

6. Enjoy the pickles as a snack or side dish. They will keep in the refrigerator for up to 2 months.

Tips:
• Use fresh, firm cucumbers for the best texture.
• You can adjust the amount of salt, sugar, or vinegar to suit your taste preferences.
• Feel free to add other spices, such as mustard seeds or red pepper flakes, for extra flavor.

31. Unsweetened applesauce

Ingredients:

• 3 lbs apples, peeled, cored, and chopped (about 8•10 medium apples)
• 1/2 cup water
• 1/2 tsp ground cinnamon (optional)

Instructions:

1. In a large saucepan, combine the chopped apples and water.

2. Bring the mixture to a boil over medium•high heat, then reduce the heat to low, cover, and simmer for 15•20 minutes, stirring occasionally, until the apples are very soft.

3. Remove the saucepan from the heat and let the apple mixture cool slightly.

4. Using a potato masher, immersion blender, or regular blender, puree the apple mixture until it reaches your desired consistency. Some texture is fine if you prefer a chunkier applesauce.

5. If using, stir in the ground cinnamon until well combined.

6. Taste the applesauce and adjust the seasoning if needed. You can add a bit more water if it's too thick.

7. Transfer the unsweetened applesauce to an airtight container and refrigerate for up to 1 week.

Tips:
• Use a variety of apples for more complex flavor.
• For a smoother texture, pass the applesauce through a fine•mesh sieve after blending.
• You can also can the applesauce for longer•term storage.

32. Grilled portobello mushrooms

Ingredients:

• 4 large portobello mushroom caps, stems removed
• 2 tbsp olive oil
• 2 tbsp balsamic vinegar
• 2 cloves garlic, minced
• 1 tsp dried thyme
• Salt and pepper to taste

Instructions:

1. Clean the portobello mushroom caps by gently wiping them with a damp paper towel to remove any dirt or debris. Remove the stems.

2. In a shallow baking dish or resealable plastic bag, combine the olive oil, balsamic vinegar, minced garlic, and dried thyme. Add the mushroom caps and toss to coat them evenly in the marinade.

3. Cover the dish or seal the bag and let the mushrooms marinate for 30 minutes to 1 hour, flipping them occasionally.

4. Preheat your grill or grill pan to medium•high heat.

5. Remove the mushrooms from the marinade and place them cap•side down on the hot grill. Grill for 4•5 minutes per side, until the mushrooms are tender and have grill marks.

6. Transfer the grilled portobello mushrooms to a serving plate. Season with salt and pepper to taste.

7. Serve the grilled portobellos as a main dish, or use them as a burger patty substitute. They also make a great side dish.

Tips:
• Brush the grill grates with oil to prevent the mushrooms from sticking.
• For extra flavor, baste the mushrooms with the leftover marinade while grilling.
• Try adding other herbs or spices to the marinade, such as rosemary, oregano, or smoked paprika.
• Grilled portobellos pair well with grilled vegetables, salads, or your favorite protein.

33. Grilled eggplant slices

Ingredients:

• 1 medium eggplant, sliced into 1/2•inch thick rounds
• 1 tbsp olive oil
• 1/4 tsp salt
• 1/8 tsp black pepper

Instructions:

1. Preheat your grill or grill pan to medium•high heat.

2. In a large bowl, toss the eggplant slices with the olive oil, salt, and pepper until evenly coated.

3. Grill the eggplant slices for 3•5 minutes per side, until they are tender and have grill marks.

4. Transfer the grilled eggplant slices to a serving plate or platter.

Benefits of Grilled Eggplant for Weight Loss:

• Very low in calories • 1 cup of grilled eggplant has only 35 calories.

• High in fiber • eggplant is a good source of dietary fiber.

• 0 points on many weight loss programs • eggplant is typically a 0 point food.

• Versatile • grilled eggplant can be enjoyed on its own or incorporated into a variety of dishes.

• Flavorful • the grilling process brings out the natural sweetness of the eggplant.

Grilled eggplant slices make a fantastic 0 point weight loss side dish or snack. You can enjoy them on their own or use them in recipes like eggplant parmesan, ratatouille, or as a topping for salads and sandwiches.

34. Steamed green beans

Ingredients:

• 1 lb fresh green beans, trimmed
• 1•2 tbsp water
• Salt and pepper to taste

Instructions:

1. Rinse the green beans and trim off the ends. Cut into 1•2 inch pieces if desired.

2. Place the green beans in a steamer basket or colander set over a pot of simmering water. Make sure the beans are not submerged in the water.

3. Cover and steam the green beans for 5•7 minutes, until tender•crisp. The timing may vary depending on the thickness of the beans.

4. Carefully remove the steamer basket or colander from the pot. Transfer the steamed green beans to a serving bowl.

5. Season the green beans with salt and pepper to taste. You can also toss them with a bit of butter, olive oil, or lemon juice if desired.

6. Serve the steamed green beans hot. Enjoy!

The key is to steam the beans just until they are tender but still have a nice bite to them. Be careful not to overcook.

35. Steamed spinach

Ingredients:

• 1 lb fresh spinach, washed and stems removed
• 1 tbsp water
• 1/4 tsp salt
• 1/8 tsp black pepper

Instructions:

1. Fill a medium saucepan with about 1 inch of water and bring it to a boil over high heat.

2. Place the washed and trimmed spinach in a steamer basket or colander that fits inside the saucepan.

3. Carefully lower the steamer basket or colander into the boiling water. Cover and steam the spinach for 2•3 minutes, until it is wilted and tender.

4. Transfer the steamed spinach to a serving bowl. Drizzle with the 1 tbsp of water and season with the salt and black pepper. Toss gently to coat.

5. Serve the steamed spinach warm.

Benefits of Steamed Spinach for Weight Loss:

• Extremely low in calories • 1 cup of steamed spinach has only 41 calories.

• High in fiber, vitamins, and minerals • spinach is a nutrient•dense superfood.

• 0 points on many weight loss programs • spinach is typically a 0 point food.

• Versatile • steamed spinach can be enjoyed on its own or incorporated into a variety of dishes.

Steamed spinach is a fantastic 0 point weight loss food that provides a wealth of nutrients and fiber to keep you feeling full and satisfied. It's a simple and delicious way to add more greens to your diet.

36. Seaweed salad

Ingredients:

- 1 oz (28g) dried wakame seaweed
- 2 tbsp rice vinegar
- 1 tbsp soy sauce
- 1 tsp sesame oil
- 1 tsp white sugar
- 1 tsp sesame seeds
- 1 green onion, thinly sliced
- 1 tsp toasted sesame seeds (for garnish)

Instructions:

1. Soak the dried wakame seaweed in water for 5•10 minutes until softened. Drain and rinse the wakame under cold water. Squeeze out any excess water and roughly chop the seaweed.

2. In a medium bowl, whisk together the rice vinegar, soy sauce, sesame oil, and sugar until the sugar has dissolved.

3. Add the chopped wakame, sesame seeds, and sliced green onion to the dressing. Toss everything together until well combined.

4. Transfer the seaweed salad to a serving bowl or plate. Sprinkle the toasted sesame seeds over the top as a garnish.

5. Chill the seaweed salad in the refrigerator for at least 30 minutes before serving to allow the flavors to meld.

Tips:
- You can use other types of seaweed, such as hijiki or arame, in place of the wakame.
- For extra crunch, add some thinly sliced cucumber or carrot.
- Adjust the amount of soy sauce, vinegar, or sugar to suit your taste preferences.
- Serve the seaweed salad as a side dish or appetizer.

This refreshing and flavorful seaweed salad is a great way to enjoy the nutritional benefits of sea vegetables. Enjoy!

37. Jicama sticks

Ingredients:

- 1 medium jicama, peeled and cut into 1/4•inch thick sticks
- 1 tbsp lime juice
- 1/4 tsp chili powder (optional)
- 1/8 tsp salt

Instructions:

1. Peel the jicama and cut it into 1/4•inch thick sticks or matchsticks.

2. In a medium bowl, toss the jicama sticks with the lime juice, chili powder (if using), and salt until evenly coated.

3. Serve the jicama sticks immediately, or refrigerate until ready to enjoy.

Benefits of Jicama Sticks for Weight Loss:

- Very low in calories • 1 cup of jicama sticks has only 45 calories.

- High in fiber • jicama is an excellent source of dietary fiber.

- 0 points on many weight loss programs • jicama is typically a 0 point food.

- Crunchy and refreshing • the crisp texture makes jicama sticks a great snack.

- Versatile • you can enjoy jicama sticks on their own or with a 0 point dip.

The lime juice and chili powder add a tasty kick to the naturally sweet and crunchy jicama. Jicama sticks make a fantastic 0 point weight loss snack that can help satisfy cravings for something crisp and flavorful.

38. Broccoli slaw (dressing made with low•fat yogurt)

Ingredients:

Slaw:
• 1 head of broccoli, stems and florets shredded or finely chopped
• 1 carrot, shredded
• 1/2 red onion, thinly sliced
• 1/4 cup sliced almonds (optional)

Yogurt Dressing:
• 1/2 cup low•fat plain Greek yogurt
• 2 tablespoons apple cider vinegar
• 1 tablespoon honey
• 1 teaspoon Dijon mustard
• 1/4 teaspoon salt
• 1/8 teaspoon black pepper

Instructions:

1. In a large bowl, combine the shredded broccoli, shredded carrot, sliced red onion, and sliced almonds (if using). Set aside.

2. In a small bowl, whisk together the yogurt, apple cider vinegar, honey, Dijon mustard, salt, and black pepper to make the dressing.

3. Pour the yogurt dressing over the broccoli slaw and toss gently to coat the vegetables evenly.

4. Cover the broccoli slaw and refrigerate for at least 30 minutes, or up to 24 hours, to allow the flavors to meld.

5. Serve the broccoli slaw chilled or at room temperature.

Tips:
• For a creamier dressing, use full•fat Greek yogurt instead of low•fat.
• Add other crunchy ingredients like sunflower seeds, pumpkin seeds, or chopped celery.
• Customize the dressing by using different types of vinegar (e.g., white wine vinegar, rice vinegar) or adding herbs like dill or parsley.
• This slaw makes a great side dish, but it can also be used as a topping for sandwiches, burgers, or tacos.
• The slaw will keep in the refrigerator for up to 5 days.

Enjoy this healthy and flavorful broccoli slaw with the tangy yogurt dressing!

39. Grilled artichokes

Ingredients:

• 4 medium artichokes
• 1/4 cup olive oil
• 2 tablespoons lemon juice
• 2 cloves garlic, minced
• 1 teaspoon dried oregano
• 1/2 teaspoon salt
• 1/4 teaspoon black pepper

For Serving:
• Lemon wedges
• Garlic aioli or other dipping sauce (optional)

Instructions:
1. Prepare the artichokes:
   • Trim the stem of each artichoke, leaving about 1 inch.
   • Using a sharp knife, cut off the top 1•2 inches of the artichoke.
   • Using kitchen shears, snip off the sharp tips of the outer leaves.
   • Rub the cut surfaces with lemon juice to prevent browning.

2. In a small bowl, whisk together the olive oil, lemon juice, garlic, oregano, salt, and pepper.

3. Place the prepared artichokes in a large bowl and pour the seasoned oil mixture over them, turning to coat evenly.

4. Preheat your grill or grill pan to medium•high heat.

5. Place the artichokes on the hot grill, cover, and cook for 12•15 minutes, turning occasionally, until the leaves are tender and can be easily pulled off.

6. Transfer the grilled artichokes to a serving platter. Serve warm, with lemon wedges and a garlic aioli or other dipping sauce, if desired.

Tips:
• You can also steam the artichokes for 15•20 minutes before grilling to help them cook through.
• For a more intense smoky flavor, grill the artichokes over direct high heat for 2•3 minutes per side before moving them to medium•high heat.
• Experiment with different herb and spice combinations in the seasoning mixture.
• Serve the grilled artichokes as an appetizer or side dish.

40. Cauliflower rice

Ingredients:

• 1 medium head of cauliflower, cut into florets
• 1 tablespoon olive oil or avocado oil (optional)
• Salt and pepper to taste

Instructions:

1. Wash and dry the cauliflower florets thoroughly.

2. Working in batches, place the cauliflower florets in a food processor and pulse until the cauliflower is broken down into small, rice•like pieces. Be careful not to over•process, as you don't want the cauliflower to become a puree.

3. Alternatively, you can grate the cauliflower florets using a box grater to create the "rice" texture.

4. (Optional) In a large skillet or wok, heat the olive oil or avocado oil over medium heat. Add the riced cauliflower and sauté for 3•5 minutes, stirring occasionally, until the cauliflower is tender and has a slightly drier texture.

5. Season the cauliflower rice with salt and pepper to taste.

Serving Suggestions:
• Use the cauliflower rice as a low•carb substitute for regular rice in dishes like stir•fries, burrito bowls, or fried rice.

• Mix the cauliflower rice with sautéed vegetables, herbs, and spices for a simple side dish.

• Bake the cauliflower rice into a casserole or use it as a base for a grain•free pizza crust.

• Freeze the raw cauliflower rice in an airtight container for up to 3 months. Thaw and use as needed.

Tips:
• Work in batches when processing the cauliflower to ensure an even, rice•like texture.
• Squeeze out any excess moisture from the riced cauliflower before cooking, if desired.
• Experiment with different seasonings, such as garlic powder, onion powder, or Italian herbs.
• For a creamier texture, stir in a bit of butter or cream cheese after cooking.

Enjoy your homemade cauliflower rice!

41. Turkey lettuce wraps

Ingredients:

- 1 lb ground turkey
- 1 tablespoon olive oil
- 1 onion, diced
- 3 cloves garlic, minced
- 1 tablespoon grated ginger
- 2 tablespoons soy sauce
- 1 tablespoon rice vinegar
- 1 teaspoon sesame oil
- 1/4 teaspoon red pepper flakes (optional)
- Salt and pepper to taste
- 1 head of lettuce (such as bibb, romaine, or butter lettuce), leaves separated

For Serving:
- Chopped green onions
- Shredded carrots
- Sliced cucumber
- Toasted sesame seeds

Instructions:

1. In a large skillet or wok, heat the olive oil over medium•high heat. Add the ground turkey and cook, breaking it up with a wooden spoon, until browned and cooked through, about 5•7 minutes.

2. Add the diced onion and cook for 2•3 minutes, until softened.

3. Stir in the minced garlic and grated ginger. Cook for 1 minute, until fragrant.

4. Add the soy sauce, rice vinegar, sesame oil, and red pepper flakes (if using). Season with salt and pepper to taste. Stir to combine.

5. Reduce the heat to low and let the turkey mixture simmer for 2•3 minutes to allow the flavors to meld.

6. To serve, place a spoonful of the turkey mixture into the center of a lettuce leaf. Top with desired toppings such as chopped green onions, shredded carrots, sliced cucumber, and toasted sesame seeds.

7. Fold the lettuce leaf around the filling and enjoy.

42. Chicken skewers (grilled with spices)

Ingredients:

• 1 lb boneless, skinless chicken breasts, cut into 1•inch cubes
• 2 tablespoons olive oil
• 2 teaspoons paprika
• 1 teaspoon garlic powder
• 1 teaspoon ground cumin
• 1/2 teaspoon chili powder
• 1/2 teaspoon salt
• 1/4 teaspoon black pepper
• Wooden or metal skewers, soaked in water for 30 minutes (if using wooden)

Instructions:

1. In a large bowl, combine the cubed chicken, olive oil, paprika, garlic powder, cumin, chili powder, salt, and black pepper. Toss to coat the chicken evenly with the spices.

2. Thread the marinated chicken cubes onto the soaked wooden skewers or metal skewers, leaving a small space between each piece.

3. Preheat your grill or grill pan to medium•high heat.

4. Grill the chicken skewers for 12•15 minutes, turning occasionally, until the chicken is cooked through and no longer pink in the center.

5. Transfer the grilled chicken skewers to a serving platter.

Serving Suggestions:
• Serve the grilled chicken skewers as an appetizer or main dish.
• Accompany the skewers with grilled vegetables, such as bell peppers, zucchini, or onions.
• Serve the chicken skewers with a side of rice, quinoa, or pita bread.
• Offer a dipping sauce, such as tzatziki, pesto, or a spicy yogurt sauce.

Tips:
• Adjust the spice blend to your taste preferences, adding more or less of the seasonings.
• Marinate the chicken for 30 minutes to 1 hour in the refrigerator for even more flavor.
• Soak wooden skewers in water for at least 30 minutes to prevent them from burning on the grill.
• Use metal skewers for easier handling and to prevent the chicken from falling off.
• Grill the skewers over direct high heat for a nice char, or move them to indirect heat if they're browning too quickly.

43. Turkey meatballs (baked)

Ingredients:

• 1 lb ground turkey
• 1/2 cup breadcrumbs
• 1/4 cup grated Parmesan cheese
• 1 egg, lightly beaten
• 2 cloves garlic, minced
• 1 tsp dried oregano
• 1/2 tsp salt
• 1/4 tsp black pepper

Instructions:

1. Preheat your oven to 400°F (200°C). Line a baking sheet with parchment paper or a silicone baking mat.

2. In a large bowl, combine the ground turkey, breadcrumbs, Parmesan cheese, egg, garlic, oregano, salt, and pepper. Mix everything together until well incorporated.

3. Using a small cookie scoop or spoon, form the mixture into 1•inch meatballs and place them on the prepared baking sheet, spacing them about 1 inch apart.

4. Bake the turkey meatballs in the preheated oven for 18•22 minutes, or until they are cooked through and no longer pink in the center.

5. Remove the baked meatballs from the oven and let them cool for a few minutes before serving.

Serving Suggestions:
• Serve the turkey meatballs as an appetizer with a dipping sauce, such as marinara or pesto.
• Add the meatballs to a pasta dish, such as spaghetti or penne.
• Use the meatballs in a meatball sub or sandwich.
• Incorporate the meatballs into a soup or stew.

Tips:
• For extra moisture and flavor, you can add a tablespoon of milk or grated onion to the meatball mixture.
• Experiment with different herbs and spices, such as basil, parsley, or red pepper flakes.
• To make the meatballs ahead of time, you can freeze them uncooked on the baking sheet, then transfer them to a freezer•safe bag or container. Bake them straight from frozen, adding a few extra minutes to the cooking time.

44. Baked tofu cubes

Ingredients:

• 1 block (14 oz) extra•firm tofu, drained and pressed
• 2 tablespoons soy sauce or tamari
• 1 tablespoon rice vinegar
• 1 tablespoon maple syrup or agave nectar
• 1 teaspoon sesame oil
• 1/2 teaspoon garlic powder
• 1/2 teaspoon ground ginger
• 1/4 teaspoon black pepper

Instructions:

1. Preheat your oven to 400°F (200°C). Line a baking sheet with parchment paper or a silicone baking mat.

2. Drain the tofu and press it between two plates or paper towels to remove excess moisture. Cut the tofu into 1•inch cubes.

3. In a medium bowl, whisk together the soy sauce, rice vinegar, maple syrup, sesame oil, garlic powder, ground ginger, and black pepper.

4. Add the tofu cubes to the marinade and gently toss to coat them evenly.

5. Arrange the marinated tofu cubes in a single layer on the prepared baking sheet.

6. Bake the tofu for 20•25 minutes, flipping the cubes halfway through, until they are golden brown and crispy on the outside. Remove the baked tofu cubes from the oven and let them cool for a few minutes before serving.

Serving Suggestions:
• Serve the baked tofu cubes as a snack or appetizer.
• Add them to salads, grain bowls, or stir•fries for extra protein.
• Toss the baked tofu cubes with your favorite sauce or dressing.
• Use the tofu cubes in vegetarian or vegan dishes.

Tips:
• Press the tofu for at least 30 minutes to remove as much moisture as possible before marinating and baking.
• Adjust the marinade ingredients to your taste preferences, adding more sweetness or spice as desired.
• For a crispier texture, toss the tofu cubes with a tablespoon of cornstarch or arrowroot powder before baking.

45. Quinoa salad (with lemon vinaigrette)

Ingredients:

Salad:
• 1 cup uncooked quinoa, rinsed
• 1 cup cherry tomatoes, halved
• 1 cucumber, diced
• 1 bell pepper, diced
• 1/2 cup crumbled feta cheese
• 1/4 cup chopped fresh parsley
• 2 tablespoons chopped fresh mint (optional)

Lemon Vinaigrette:
• 3 tablespoons olive oil
• 2 tablespoons lemon juice
• 1 tablespoon white wine vinegar
• 1 teaspoon Dijon mustard
• 1 garlic clove, minced
• 1/2 teaspoon salt
• 1/4 teaspoon black pepper

Instructions:
1. Cook the quinoa according to package instructions. Fluff with a fork and let cool.

2. In a large bowl, combine the cooked quinoa, cherry tomatoes, cucumber, bell pepper, feta cheese, parsley, and mint (if using).

3. In a small bowl, whisk together the olive oil, lemon juice, white wine vinegar, Dijon mustard, garlic, salt, and pepper to make the lemon vinaigrette.

4. Pour the lemon vinaigrette over the quinoa salad and toss gently to coat. Refrigerate the quinoa salad for at least 30 minutes to allow the flavors to meld. Serve chilled or at room temperature.

Tips:
• Use a variety of colorful vegetables for a visually appealing salad.
• Swap out the feta for another cheese, such as goat cheese or shredded mozzarella.
• Add in other mix•ins like chickpeas, olives, or toasted nuts.
• For a heartier meal, top the salad with grilled chicken or shrimp.
• The salad can be made a day in advance and stored in the refrigerator.

46. Lentil soup (low•sodium)

Ingredients:

• 1 cup dry brown or green lentils, rinsed
• 6 cups low•sodium vegetable or chicken broth
• 1 onion, diced
• 2 carrots, peeled and diced
• 2 celery stalks, diced
• 3 garlic cloves, minced
• 1 teaspoon dried thyme
• 1 bay leaf
• 1/4 teaspoon black pepper
• 2 cups chopped kale or spinach (optional)
• Lemon wedges for serving (optional)

Instructions:
1. In a large pot, combine the rinsed lentils and broth. Bring to a boil over high heat.

2. Reduce the heat to medium•low, cover, and simmer for 15•20 minutes, or until the lentils are tender.

3. Add the diced onion, carrots, celery, and garlic to the pot. Stir in the dried thyme and bay leaf. Season with black pepper.

4. Continue simmering the soup, uncovered, for an additional 15•20 minutes, or until the vegetables are tender.

5. If using, stir in the chopped kale or spinach and cook for 5 more minutes until the greens are wilted.

6. Taste the soup and adjust seasoning if needed. Remove the bay leaf before serving. Serve the low•sodium lentil soup warm, with a squeeze of lemon juice if desired.

Nutritional Information (per serving):
• Calories: 200
• Total Fat: 1g
• Saturated Fat: 0g
• Sodium: 150mg
• Carbohydrates: 35g
• Fiber: 12g
• Protein: 12g

47. Black bean soup (low•sodium)

Ingredients:

• 2 cans (15 oz each) low•sodium black beans, rinsed and drained
• 4 cups low•sodium vegetable or chicken broth
• 1 onion, diced
• 2 carrots, peeled and diced
• 2 celery stalks, diced
• 3 garlic cloves, minced
• 1 teaspoon ground cumin
• 1 teaspoon dried oregano
• 1/4 teaspoon chili powder
• 1/4 teaspoon black pepper
• Chopped fresh cilantro for garnish (optional)
• Lime wedges for serving (optional)

Instructions:

1. In a large pot, combine the rinsed and drained black beans and the low•sodium broth. Bring the mixture to a boil over high heat.

2. Reduce the heat to medium•low and add the diced onion, carrots, celery, and garlic. Stir in the ground cumin, dried oregano, chili powder, and black pepper.

3. Simmer the soup, uncovered, for 20•25 minutes, stirring occasionally, until the vegetables are tender.

4. Using an immersion blender or a regular blender, puree about half of the soup to create a creamy texture. (Be careful when blending hot liquids.)

5. Return the pureed portion to the pot and stir to combine. Taste the soup and adjust seasoning if needed. Serve the low•sodium black bean soup warm, garnished with chopped fresh cilantro if desired. Offer lime wedges on the side.

Nutritional Information (per serving):
• Calories: 180
• Total Fat: 1g
• Saturated Fat: 0g
• Sodium: 150mg
• Carbohydrates: 32g
• Fiber: 10g
• Protein: 10g

48. Minestrone soup (vegetable•based)

Ingredients:

• 2 tablespoons olive oil
• 1 onion, diced
• 3 carrots, peeled and diced
• 3 celery stalks, diced
• 3 garlic cloves, minced
• 1 zucchini, diced
• 1 (15 oz) can diced tomatoes
• 1 (15 oz) can kidney beans, rinsed and drained
• 4 cups low•sodium vegetable broth
• 1 cup small pasta (such as ditalini or elbow macaroni)
• 1 teaspoon dried oregano
• 1 teaspoon dried basil
• 1/4 teaspoon red pepper flakes (optional)
• Salt and black pepper to taste
• Grated Parmesan cheese for serving (optional)
• Chopped fresh parsley for garnish (optional)

Instructions:

1. In a large pot or Dutch oven, heat the olive oil over medium heat. Add the diced onion, carrots, celery, and garlic. Sauté for 5•7 minutes, until the vegetables are softened.

2. Stir in the diced zucchini and cook for an additional 2•3 minutes.

3. Add the diced tomatoes, kidney beans, vegetable broth, pasta, dried oregano, dried basil, and red pepper flakes (if using). Season with salt and black pepper to taste.

4. Bring the soup to a boil, then reduce the heat and let it simmer for 15•20 minutes, or until the pasta is tender.

5. Taste the soup and adjust seasoning if needed. Serve the vegetable minestrone soup hot, garnished with grated Parmesan cheese and chopped fresh parsley, if desired.

Nutritional Information (per serving):
• Calories: 250
• Total Fat: 5g
• Saturated Fat: 1g
• Sodium: 350mg
• Carbohydrates: 40g
• Fiber: 8g

49. Gazpacho

Ingredients:

• 4 large tomatoes, diced
• 1 cucumber, peeled, seeded, and diced
• 1 red bell pepper, diced
• 1 small red onion, diced
• 2 garlic cloves, minced
• 2 tablespoons red wine vinegar
• 1 tablespoon olive oil
• 1 teaspoon Dijon mustard
• 1/4 cup chopped fresh basil
• 1/4 cup chopped fresh parsley
• 1 cup low•sodium vegetable or tomato juice
• Salt and black pepper to taste

Instructions:

1. In a large bowl, combine the diced tomatoes, cucumber, bell pepper, red onion, and garlic.

2. In a small bowl, whisk together the red wine vinegar, olive oil, and Dijon mustard. Pour the dressing over the vegetable mixture and toss to coat.

3. Stir in the chopped basil and parsley.

4. Add the vegetable or tomato juice and season with salt and black pepper to taste.

5. Cover the gazpacho and refrigerate for at least 2 hours, or up to 24 hours, to allow the flavors to meld.

6. Serve the chilled gazpacho in bowls or glasses, garnished with additional basil or parsley if desired.

Nutritional Information (per serving):
• Calories: 100
• Total Fat: 4g
• Saturated Fat: 0.5g
• Sodium: 150mg
• Carbohydrates: 12g
• Fiber: 3g
• Protein: 3g

50. Ratatouille

Ingredients:

• 2 tablespoons olive oil
• 1 medium eggplant, cut into 1•inch cubes
• 1 medium zucchini, sliced into 1/2•inch rounds
• 1 medium yellow squash, sliced into 1/2•inch rounds
• 1 red bell pepper, seeded and cut into 1•inch pieces
• 1 onion, diced
• 3 garlic cloves, minced
• 1 (14.5 oz) can diced tomatoes
• 2 tablespoons tomato paste
• 1 teaspoon dried thyme
• 1 teaspoon dried oregano
• Salt and freshly ground black pepper to taste
• 2 tablespoons chopped fresh basil

Instructions:

1. In a large skillet or Dutch oven, heat the olive oil over medium•high heat. Add the eggplant, zucchini, yellow squash, and bell pepper. Cook, stirring occasionally, until the vegetables are starting to soften, about 5•7 minutes.

2. Add the onion and garlic to the pan. Cook for 2•3 minutes, until the onion is translucent.

3. Stir in the diced tomatoes, tomato paste, thyme, and oregano. Season with salt and pepper to taste.

4. Reduce the heat to medium•low and let the ratatouille simmer, stirring occasionally, for 20•25 minutes, until the vegetables are very tender.

5. Remove from heat and stir in the chopped fresh basil.

6. Serve the ratatouille warm, either as a main dish or as a side. It's delicious on its own or served over pasta, rice, or crusty bread.

Tips:
• Try to use a variety of colorful vegetables for the best presentation.
• Adjust the cooking time if your vegetables are cut into larger or smaller pieces.
• Add a splash of red wine or balsamic vinegar for extra flavor.
• Top with grated Parmesan cheese or crumbled feta if desired.

51. Roasted garlic mushrooms

Ingredients:

• 1 lb cremini or button mushrooms, cleaned and halved or quartered if large
• 3 tablespoons olive oil
• 4 cloves garlic, minced
• 1 teaspoon dried thyme
• 1/2 teaspoon salt
• 1/4 teaspoon black pepper
• 2 tablespoons chopped fresh parsley (optional)

Instructions:

1. Preheat your oven to 400°F (200°C). Line a baking sheet with parchment paper or a silicone baking mat.

2. In a large bowl, toss the cleaned and halved/quartered mushrooms with the olive oil, minced garlic, dried thyme, salt, and black pepper until the mushrooms are evenly coated.

3. Spread the seasoned mushrooms in a single layer on the prepared baking sheet.

4. Roast the mushrooms in the preheated oven for 20•25 minutes, stirring halfway, until they are tender and lightly browned.

5. Remove the roasted garlic mushrooms from the oven and transfer them to a serving bowl.

6. If using, sprinkle the chopped fresh parsley over the roasted mushrooms and toss to combine.

7. Serve the roasted garlic mushrooms warm, as a side dish or appetizer.

Tips:
• For even cooking, make sure the mushrooms are in a single layer on the baking sheet.
• Adjust the roasting time based on the size and type of mushrooms you're using. Larger or denser mushrooms may need a few extra minutes.
• Try using a mix of mushroom varieties, such as cremini, shiitake, and oyster, for more complex flavor.
• Add a splash of balsamic vinegar or lemon juice to the roasted mushrooms for a touch of acidity.
• Serve the roasted garlic mushrooms over pasta, rice, or mashed potatoes for a heartier meal.

52. Roasted cherry tomatoes

Ingredients:

• 1 lb cherry or grape tomatoes, halved
• 2 tablespoons olive oil
• 2 cloves garlic, minced
• 1 teaspoon dried oregano
• 1/2 teaspoon salt
• 1/4 teaspoon black pepper
• 2 tablespoons fresh basil, chopped (optional)

Instructions:

1. Preheat your oven to 400°F (200°C).

2. In a large bowl, combine the halved cherry tomatoes, olive oil, minced garlic, dried oregano, salt, and black pepper. Toss everything together until the tomatoes are evenly coated.

3. Spread the seasoned tomatoes in a single layer on a large baking sheet lined with parchment paper or a silicone baking mat.

4. Roast the tomatoes in the preheated oven for 20•25 minutes, or until they are softened and starting to burst.

5. Remove the roasted cherry tomatoes from the oven and let them cool for a few minutes.

6. Transfer the roasted tomatoes to a serving bowl and stir in the chopped fresh basil, if using.

7. Serve the roasted cherry tomatoes warm or at room temperature. They make a great side dish or can be used in salads, pasta dishes, or as a topping for bruschetta.

Tips:
• For best results, use fresh, ripe cherry or grape tomatoes.
• Adjust the roasting time based on the size of your tomatoes • larger ones may need a few extra minutes.
• Try adding other herbs or spices, such as thyme, rosemary, or red pepper flakes, to the seasoning mix.
• Roast the tomatoes at a higher temperature (425°F) for a more caramelized, intense flavor.

53. Baked apple slices (with cinnamon)

Ingredients:

• 3 medium apples, cored and sliced into 1/4•inch thick rounds
• 1 teaspoon ground cinnamon
• 1/4 teaspoon ground nutmeg (optional)
• Pinch of salt

Instructions:

1. Preheat your oven to 375°F (190°C). Line a baking sheet with parchment paper or a silicone baking mat.

2. In a large bowl, toss the apple slices with the ground cinnamon, nutmeg (if using), and a pinch of salt until the apples are evenly coated.

3. Arrange the cinnamon•coated apple slices in a single layer on the prepared baking sheet.

4. Bake the apple slices in the preheated oven for 20•25 minutes, flipping them halfway, until they are tender and lightly browned.

5. Remove the baked apple slices from the oven and let them cool for a few minutes before serving.

Nutritional Information (per serving, about 1/2 cup):
• Calories: 50
• Total Fat: 0g
• Saturated Fat: 0g
• Sodium: 5mg
• Carbohydrates: 13g
• Fiber: 2g
• Protein: 0g

Tips:
• Choose firm, crisp apples like Honeycrisp, Gala, or Fuji for the best texture.
• Adjust the baking time based on the thickness of your apple slices. Thinner slices may cook faster.
• For a sweeter flavor, you can drizzle a small amount of honey or maple syrup over the apple slices before baking.
• Serve the baked apple slices warm or at room temperature as a snack or dessert.
• These apple slices also make a great topping for oatmeal, yogurt, or ice cream.

54. Poached pear

Ingredients:

• 4 ripe but firm pears, peeled, halved, and cored
• 2 cups red wine (or apple juice for a non•alcoholic version)
• 1/2 cup granulated sugar
• 1 cinnamon stick
• 3 whole cloves
• 1 vanilla bean, split lengthwise (or 1 tsp vanilla extract)
• Juice of 1 lemon

Instructions:
1. In a large saucepan, combine the red wine (or apple juice), sugar, cinnamon stick, cloves, and vanilla bean (or vanilla extract). Bring the mixture to a simmer over medium heat, stirring occasionally until the sugar has dissolved.

2. Carefully add the peeled, halved, and cored pear halves to the simmering liquid. Squeeze the lemon juice over the pears.

3. Reduce the heat to low, cover the saucepan, and let the pears poach for 20•30 minutes, or until they are tender when pierced with a fork.

4. Using a slotted spoon, transfer the poached pear halves to a serving dish.

5. Increase the heat and let the poaching liquid simmer for 5•10 minutes, or until it has reduced and thickened slightly.

6. Pour the reduced poaching liquid over the pear halves.

7. Serve the poached pears warm or chilled, with the reduced poaching liquid spooned over the top.

Nutritional Information (per serving, 1 pear half):
• Calories: 120
• Total Fat: 0g
• Saturated Fat: 0g
• Sodium: 0mg
• Carbohydrates: 25g
• Fiber: 4g
• Protein: 1g

55. Grilled peaches

Ingredients:

- 4 ripe but firm peaches, halved and pitted
- 2 tablespoons olive oil or melted butter
- 2 tablespoons brown sugar (optional)
- Vanilla ice cream or whipped cream (optional, for serving)

Instructions:

1. Preheat your grill or grill pan to medium•high heat.

2. Brush the cut sides of the peach halves with the olive oil or melted butter.

3. If using, sprinkle the brown sugar evenly over the cut sides of the peaches.

4. Place the peach halves, cut•side down, directly on the grill grates. Grill for 3•5 minutes, until grill marks appear and the peaches start to soften.

5. Carefully flip the peach halves over and grill for an additional 2•3 minutes, until the peaches are tender but still hold their shape.

6. Remove the grilled peaches from the grill and transfer to a serving plate.

7. Serve the grilled peaches warm, either on their own or with a scoop of vanilla ice cream or a dollop of whipped cream, if desired.

Tips:
- Choose ripe but firm peaches for the best texture when grilled.

- Adjust the grilling time based on the ripeness of your peaches • riper peaches will cook faster.

- For extra flavor, brush the peaches with a bit of honey or maple syrup before grilling.

- Try adding a sprinkle of cinnamon or a drizzle of balsamic glaze to the grilled peaches.

- Grilled peaches also make a great topping for salads, yogurt, or oatmeal.

Enjoy these sweet and smoky grilled peaches!

56. Berry salad (with mixed berries)

Ingredients:

• 1 cup fresh strawberries, hulled and halved
• 1 cup fresh blueberries
• 1 cup fresh raspberries
• 1 cup fresh blackberries
• 1 tablespoon honey (optional)
• 1 tablespoon fresh lemon juice
• 1 tablespoon chopped fresh mint (optional)

Instructions:

1. In a large bowl, gently combine the strawberries, blueberries, raspberries, and blackberries.

2. If desired, drizzle the honey and lemon juice over the berries and toss gently to coat.

3. Sprinkle the chopped fresh mint over the berry salad, if using.

4. Serve the mixed berry salad chilled or at room temperature.

Nutritional Information (per serving, about 1 cup):
• Calories: 60
• Total Fat: 0g
• Saturated Fat: 0g
• Sodium: 0mg
• Carbohydrates: 15g
• Fiber: 4g
• Protein: 1g

Tips:
• Use a variety of fresh, in•season berries for the best flavor and texture.
• Adjust the amount of honey based on the sweetness of the berries and your personal preference.
• For a creamier texture, serve the berry salad with a dollop of plain Greek yogurt or a sprinkle of toasted nuts or seeds.
• Add a splash of balsamic glaze or a squeeze of orange juice for a touch of acidity.
• This berry salad is a great topping for oatmeal, pancakes, or waffles.
• Store any leftover berry salad in an airtight container in the refrigerator for up to 3 days.

57. Watermelon cubes

Ingredients:

• 1 small watermelon
• Optional: lime wedges for serving

Instructions:

1. Wash the watermelon and cut it in half lengthwise. Scoop out the seeds.

2. Cut the watermelon flesh into 1•inch cubes, discarding any remaining seeds as you go.

3. Transfer the watermelon cubes to a serving bowl or plate.

4. Serve the watermelon cubes chilled, with lime wedges on the side if desired. The lime juice provides a nice contrast to the sweetness of the watermelon.

That's it! Watermelon cubes make a refreshing and hydrating snack or side dish, especially on a hot day. You can also use the cubes in fruit salads, smoothies, or as a topping for yogurt or ice cream. Enjoy!

58. Cantaloupe slices

Ingredients:

• 1 cantaloupe

Instructions:

1. Wash the cantaloupe and slice it in half lengthwise. Scoop out and discard the seeds.

2. Use a sharp knife to slice the cantaloupe flesh into 1/2•inch thick slices.

3. Arrange the cantaloupe slices on a serving platter or in an airtight container.

4. Refrigerate the cantaloupe slices until ready to serve, up to 5 days.

That's it! Cantaloupe slices make a refreshing and juicy snack or side dish.

Cantaloupe is an excellent source of vitamins A and C, as well as minerals like potassium. It's also high in water content, which can help keep you hydrated.

You can enjoy the cantaloupe slices on their own, or try topping them with a sprinkle of lime juice, mint, or a drizzle of honey for extra flavor. Cantaloupe also pairs well with other fruits like berries, pineapple, or grapes in a fruit salad.

For a fun presentation, you can serve the cantaloupe slices in the hollowed•out cantaloupe rind. This makes a beautiful and edible serving bowl.

Cantaloupe slices are a refreshing and healthy snack that's perfect for hot summer days. Enjoy!

59. Honeydew melon balls

Ingredients:

• 1 small honeydew melon

Instructions:

1. Wash the honeydew melon and cut it in half lengthwise. Scoop out and discard the seeds.

2. Use a melon baller or small spoon to scoop out round balls of the honeydew flesh.

3. Transfer the melon balls to a serving bowl or airtight container.

4. Refrigerate the melon balls until ready to serve, up to 5 days.

That's it! Honeydew melon balls make a refreshing, hydrating, and low•calorie snack. They have 0 Weight Watchers points, making them an excellent choice for weight loss.

You can enjoy the melon balls on their own, or try adding them to fruit salads, yogurt parfaits, or even cocktails. The sweet, juicy flavor pairs well with other fruits like grapes, pineapple, or berries.

Honeydew melon is a great source of vitamins A, C, and B6, as well as minerals like potassium. It's also high in water content, which can help keep you feeling full and hydrated.

For a fun presentation, you can serve the melon balls in the hollowed•out honeydew rind. This makes a beautiful and edible serving bowl. Enjoy this healthy, 0 point snack!

60. Pineapple chunks

Ingredients:

• 1 fresh pineapple

Instructions:

1. Wash the pineapple and cut off the top and bottom ends.

2. Stand the pineapple upright on a cutting board. Using a sharp knife, carefully slice off the outer rind, removing all the eyes and skin.

3. Once the pineapple is peeled, cut it in half lengthwise. Use a knife or melon baller to cut the pineapple flesh into 1•inch cubes or chunks.

4. Transfer the pineapple chunks to a serving bowl or airtight container.

5. Refrigerate the pineapple chunks until ready to serve, up to 5 days.

That's it! Pineapple chunks make a refreshing and juicy snack or addition to fruit salads. They are packed with vitamin C, manganese, and bromelain, an enzyme that can aid digestion.

You can enjoy the pineapple chunks on their own, or try pairing them with other tropical fruits like mango, kiwi, or papaya. They also make a great topping for yogurt, oatmeal, or even grilled meats and fish.

For a fun presentation, you can thread the pineapple chunks onto skewers for a colorful and portable snack. Pineapple chunks are a versatile and healthy treat that everyone will love.

61. Mango slices

Ingredients:

• 1•2 ripe mangoes

Instructions:

1. Wash the mangoes and slice them in half lengthwise, cutting around the large flat pit in the center.

2. Use a sharp knife to carefully slice the mango flesh into 1/2•inch thick slices.

3. Arrange the mango slices in a single layer on a plate or in an airtight container.

4. Refrigerate the mango slices until ready to serve, up to 5 days.

That's it! Mango slices make a sweet, juicy, and refreshing snack or addition to fruit salads.

Mangoes are an excellent source of vitamins A and C, as well as fiber and antioxidants. They have a bright, tropical flavor that pairs well with other fruits like pineapple, kiwi, or berries.

You can enjoy the mango slices on their own, or try drizzling them with a bit of lime juice or honey for extra flavor. They also make a great topping for yogurt, oatmeal, or even grilled fish or chicken.

For a fun presentation, you can fan the mango slices out on a plate or platter. You can also thread them onto skewers for a portable snack.

Mango slices are a delicious and nutritious way to enjoy this popular tropical fruit. Refrigerate them for a refreshing and healthy treat anytime!

62. Kiwi slices

Ingredients:

• 2•3 kiwi fruits

Instructions:

1. Wash the kiwi fruits and slice them into rounds about 1/4•inch thick.

2. Arrange the kiwi slices in a single layer on a plate or in an airtight container.

3. Refrigerate the kiwi slices until ready to serve, up to 5 days.

That's it! Kiwi slices make a refreshing, sweet, and tangy snack that is perfect for weight loss.

Kiwi is an excellent source of vitamin C, as well as fiber, potassium, and antioxidants. It has a low calorie count, with only about 42 calories per medium kiwi fruit. This makes kiwi slices a 0 point snack on Weight Watchers.

You can enjoy the kiwi slices on their own as a healthy snack. They also pair well with other fruits like berries, pineapple, or melon. Try adding them to yogurt, oatmeal, or salads for extra flavor and nutrition.

For a fun twist, you can also skewer the kiwi slices onto toothpicks or small wooden skewers for a colorful and portable snack.

Kiwi is a great source of fiber, which can help keep you feeling full and satisfied. Enjoy this tasty, 0 point weight loss snack!

63. Pomegranate seeds

Ingredients:

• 1 pomegranate

Instructions:

1. Cut the pomegranate in half horizontally.

2. Hold one half over a bowl, seeds facing down, and gently tap the back of the pomegranate half with a wooden spoon. The seeds should fall out into the bowl.

3. Repeat with the other half of the pomegranate.

4. Pick out any remaining white membrane pieces from the seeds.

That's it! Pomegranate seeds make a great snack on their own. They are packed with nutrients like fiber, vitamins C and K, and antioxidants. Plus, they have 0 Weight Watchers points, making them an excellent choice for weight loss.

You can enjoy the pomegranate seeds as is, or try sprinkling them on top of yogurt, salads, oatmeal, or other healthy dishes. The sweet•tart flavor and crunchy texture adds a nice pop of freshness.

Pomegranate seeds are also easy to store. Keep them refrigerated in an airtight container for up to 5 days. Enjoy this healthy, 0 point snack!

64. Steamed mussels

Ingredients:

• 2 lbs fresh mussels, scrubbed and debearded
• 1/2 cup dry white wine or seafood stock
• 2 tbsp unsalted butter
• 2 cloves garlic, minced
• 1 shallot, thinly sliced
• 1 tbsp chopped parsley
• Salt and pepper to taste
• Lemon wedges for serving

Instructions:

1. In a large pot or Dutch oven, combine the white wine or stock, butter, garlic, and shallot. Bring the liquid to a simmer over medium heat.

2. Add the cleaned mussels to the pot. Cover and steam for 5•7 minutes, until the mussels have opened up.

3. Discard any mussels that did not open. Transfer the steamed mussels to a serving bowl.

4. Sprinkle the chopped parsley over the mussels and season with salt and pepper to taste.

5. Serve the steamed mussels immediately, with lemon wedges on the side for squeezing over the top.

This steamed mussels recipe makes a delicious and easy seafood dish. Mussels are an excellent source of lean protein, vitamins, and minerals.

The white wine or stock, garlic, and shallot create a flavorful broth that the mussels steam in. The parsley adds a fresh, herbal note.

Be sure to discard any mussels that do not open, as they may be unsafe to eat. Serve the steamed mussels with crusty bread for dipping in the broth.

You can also try adding other aromatics like diced tomatoes, fennel, or saffron to the broth for extra flavor. Steamed mussels pair well with a crisp white wine or a light salad.

Enjoy this simple yet elegant steamed mussels dish as an appetizer or light main course.

65. Steamed clams

Ingredients:

- 1 lb fresh clams, scrubbed clean
- 1/2 cup dry white wine or clam juice
- 2 tbsp lemon juice
- 2 cloves garlic, minced
- 1 tbsp chopped parsley
- Salt and pepper to taste

Instructions:

1. In a large pot or Dutch oven, combine the clams, white wine or clam juice, lemon juice, and garlic.

2. Cover the pot and bring the liquid to a boil over high heat. Once boiling, reduce the heat to medium•low and steam the clams for 5•7 minutes, until they have all opened up.

3. Discard any clams that did not open. Transfer the steamed clams to a serving bowl.

4. Sprinkle the chopped parsley over the clams and season with salt and pepper to taste.

5. Serve the steamed clams immediately, with the cooking liquid spooned over the top.

This steamed clams recipe is a 0 point dish on Weight Watchers. Clams are low in calories and high in protein, making them an excellent choice for weight loss.

The white wine or clam juice, lemon juice, and garlic provide tons of flavor without adding any extra calories or points. Parsley adds a fresh, herbal note.

Serve the steamed clams as an appetizer or light main course. They pair well with crusty bread for dipping in the flavorful broth. You can also add the clams to pasta dishes, salads, or risottos.

Enjoy this healthy, 0 point weight loss recipe for steamed clams!

66. Steamed lobster tail

Ingredients:

• 2 lobster tails, thawed if frozen
• 1/2 cup water or white wine
• 1 tbsp lemon juice
• 1 tbsp butter, melted (optional)
• Salt and pepper to taste

Instructions:

1. Fill a large pot with about 1 inch of water or white wine. Bring to a boil over high heat.

2. Using kitchen shears, cut along the underside of each lobster tail to split it in half lengthwise, leaving the shell intact.

3. Place the lobster tails, cut•side up, in a steamer basket or colander. Lower the basket into the boiling liquid, making sure the tails are not submerged.

4. Cover the pot and steam the lobster tails for 8•12 minutes, until the meat is opaque and cooked through.

5. Transfer the steamed lobster tails to a serving plate. Drizzle with the melted butter and a squeeze of lemon juice.

6. Season with salt and pepper to taste.

Serve the steamed lobster tails immediately, with extra lemon wedges on the side. The sweet, tender meat pairs beautifully with the bright lemon and rich butter.

You can also serve the steamed lobster tails chilled, perhaps over a salad or with a dipping sauce like cocktail sauce or garlic butter. Enjoy this elegant and delicious seafood dish!

67. Smoked salmon

Ingredients:

- 4 oz sliced smoked salmon
- 1 tbsp cream cheese (optional)
- 1 tbsp capers (optional)
- 1 tbsp chopped dill (optional)
- Lemon wedges for serving

Instructions:

1. Arrange the sliced smoked salmon on a plate or platter.

2. If desired, top the salmon with small dollops of cream cheese, capers, and chopped dill.

3. Serve the smoked salmon immediately, with lemon wedges on the side.

That's it! Smoked salmon is a delicious and nutritious way to enjoy this flavorful fish.

Smoked salmon is an excellent source of protein, healthy fats, and important vitamins and minerals like vitamin B12, vitamin D, and omega•3 fatty acids. It makes a great addition to a weight loss diet.

The cream cheese, capers, and dill are all optional toppings that can add extra flavor and creaminess to the salmon. However, the salmon is delicious on its own as well.

You can serve the smoked salmon as an appetizer, on top of bagels or toast, or as part of a larger meal like a salad or grain bowl. It also makes a great snack when paired with crackers or cucumber slices.

Smoked salmon is a versatile and nutritious ingredient that can be enjoyed in many different ways. Enjoy this simple recipe for a delicious and healthy treat!

68. Ceviche (with lime juice)

Ingredients:

• 1 lb fresh white fish (such as tilapia, halibut, or sea bass), cut into 1/2•inch cubes
• 1 cup fresh lime juice (about 8•10 limes)
• 1/2 red onion, thinly sliced
• 1 jalapeño, seeded and minced
• 1 tomato, diced
• 1/4 cup chopped cilantro
• Salt and pepper to taste

Instructions:

1. In a large non•reactive bowl (glass or stainless steel), combine the cubed fish and lime juice. Make sure the fish is completely submerged in the lime juice.

2. Cover and refrigerate for 30 minutes to 1 hour, stirring occasionally, until the fish is opaque and "cooked" through the acid in the lime juice.

3. Drain any excess lime juice from the fish. Add the sliced red onion, minced jalapeño, diced tomato, and chopped cilantro. Gently toss to combine.

4. Season with salt and pepper to taste.

5. Serve the ceviche chilled, with tortilla chips, tostadas, or lettuce cups on the side.

The key to great ceviche is using the freshest, highest quality fish you can find. The lime juice "cooks" the fish, giving it a firm, opaque texture. Adjust the amount of jalapeño to your desired spice level. Enjoy this bright, refreshing seafood dish!

69. Tuna tartare

Ingredients:

• 8 oz sushi•grade tuna, finely diced
• 1 tbsp soy sauce
• 1 tbsp sesame oil
• 1 tbsp rice vinegar
• 1 tsp sesame seeds
• 1 tsp minced ginger
• 1 tsp minced scallions
• 1/2 tsp sriracha or other hot sauce (optional)
• Salt and pepper to taste
• Wonton chips or crackers, for serving

Instructions:

1. In a medium bowl, gently mix together the diced tuna, soy sauce, sesame oil, rice vinegar, sesame seeds, ginger, scallions, and sriracha (if using). Season with salt and pepper to taste.

2. Cover and refrigerate the tuna tartare for at least 30 minutes, up to 2 hours, to allow the flavors to meld.

3. When ready to serve, spoon the tuna tartare onto small plates or into wonton cups.

4. Serve the tuna tartare immediately, with wonton chips or crackers on the side for scooping.

Tuna tartare is a delicious and elegant raw fish dish that makes a great appetizer or light main course. The key is to use the freshest, sushi•grade tuna you can find.

The simple dressing of soy sauce, sesame oil, rice vinegar, and aromatics like ginger and scallions complements the natural flavor of the tuna without overpowering it. The sriracha adds a nice kick of heat, if desired.

Tuna is an excellent source of lean protein, healthy fats, and important nutrients like vitamin B12 and selenium. This tuna tartare recipe is a great option for a low•calorie, nutrient•dense meal or snack.

Serve the tuna tartare as an appetizer with wonton chips or crackers. You can also top it on salads, rice bowls, or avocado halves for a more substantial dish. Enjoy this fresh and flavorful tuna tartare!

70. Shrimp ceviche

Ingredients:

• 1 lb raw shrimp, peeled, deveined and diced
• 1 cup fresh lime juice (about 6•8 limes)
• 1/2 red onion, finely diced
• 1 jalapeño, seeded and minced
• 1 tomato, diced
• 1/4 cup chopped cilantro
• Salt and pepper to taste

Instructions:

1. In a large non•reactive bowl, combine the diced raw shrimp and lime juice. Stir to coat the shrimp evenly.

2. Cover and refrigerate for 30•60 minutes, stirring occasionally, until the shrimp is opaque and "cooked" through the acid in the lime juice.

3. Drain any excess lime juice from the shrimp. Add the diced red onion, minced jalapeño, diced tomato, and chopped cilantro. Gently toss to combine.

4. Season the shrimp ceviche with salt and pepper to taste.

5. Serve chilled, with lettuce cups, tostadas, or tortilla chips on the side.

This shrimp ceviche is a 0 point dish on Weight Watchers. The shrimp provides lean protein, while the lime juice, vegetables, and herbs add tons of flavor without any extra calories or points.

The acid in the lime juice "cooks" the raw shrimp, giving it a firm, opaque texture. You can adjust the amount of jalapeño to control the spice level.

Shrimp ceviche makes a refreshing and light appetizer or main course. It's packed with nutrients and perfect for weight loss. Enjoy this healthy, 0 point recipe!

71. Grilled calamari

Ingredients:

- 1 lb fresh calamari, cleaned and cut into rings
- 1 tbsp olive oil
- 1 lemon, cut into wedges
- Salt and pepper to taste

Instructions:

1. Preheat your grill or grill pan to medium•high heat.

2. In a large bowl, toss the calamari rings with the olive oil and season with a pinch of salt and pepper.

3. Grill the calamari for 2•3 minutes per side, until lightly charred and cooked through. Be careful not to overcook.

4. Transfer the grilled calamari to a serving platter. Serve immediately with lemon wedges on the side.

This grilled calamari recipe is a 0 point dish on Weight Watchers. Calamari is a lean, low•calorie seafood that is high in protein and low in carbs, making it an excellent choice for weight loss.

The simple seasoning of just olive oil, salt, and pepper allows the natural flavor of the calamari to shine. The lemon wedges provide a bright, acidic contrast that complements the slightly sweet and briny taste of the grilled calamari.

You can serve the grilled calamari as an appetizer or light main course. It pairs well with a fresh salad, roasted vegetables, or crusty bread. For extra flavor, you can also try adding a sprinkle of lemon zest, chopped parsley, or a drizzle of balsamic glaze.

Calamari is a sustainable and affordable seafood option that is packed with nutrients. Enjoy this easy, 0 point weight loss recipe for delicious grilled calamari!

72. Grilled sardines

Ingredients:

• 8•10 fresh sardines, cleaned and butterflied
• 1 tbsp olive oil
• 1 lemon, cut into wedges
• Salt and pepper to taste

Instructions:

1. Preheat your grill or grill pan to medium•high heat.

2. Rinse the sardines under cold water and pat them dry with paper towels. Use a sharp knife to butterfly the sardines by cutting along the belly and opening them up flat.

3. Brush the sardines lightly with olive oil and season both sides with salt and pepper.

4. Grill the sardines for 2•3 minutes per side, until they are lightly charred and cooked through.

5. Transfer the grilled sardines to a serving plate. Serve immediately with lemon wedges on the side.

This grilled sardines recipe is a 0 point dish on Weight Watchers. Sardines are an excellent source of lean protein, healthy fats, and essential vitamins and minerals.

The simple seasoning of just olive oil, salt, and pepper allows the natural flavor of the sardines to shine. The lemon wedges provide a bright, acidic contrast that complements the oily fish.

Sardines are a sustainable and affordable seafood option that are packed with omega•3 fatty acids. They are low in mercury and calories, making them a great choice for weight loss.

You can serve the grilled sardines as a main course with a side salad or roasted vegetables. They also make a tasty appetizer or snack when paired with crusty bread or crackers.

Enjoy this delicious and nutritious 0 point weight loss recipe for grilled sardines!

73. Pan•seared scallops

Ingredients:

- 1 lb sea scallops, patted dry
- 1 tsp olive oil
- Salt and pepper to taste
- Lemon wedges for serving

Instructions:

1. Pat the scallops very dry with paper towels. This will help them sear properly.

2. Season the scallops all over with a pinch of salt and pepper.

3. Heat a large non•stick skillet over high heat. Add the olive oil and swirl to coat the bottom of the pan.

4. Working in batches if needed, add the scallops to the hot pan in a single layer, making sure not to crowd them.

5. Sear the scallops for 2•3 minutes per side, until they develop a nice golden•brown crust and are opaque in the center.

6. Transfer the seared scallops to a plate. Repeat with any remaining scallops.

7. Serve the pan•seared scallops immediately, with lemon wedges on the side for squeezing over the top.

This pan•seared scallops recipe is a 0 point dish on Weight Watchers. Scallops are an excellent source of lean protein that is low in calories and carbs.

The high•heat searing technique cooks the scallops quickly, locking in their sweet, delicate flavor. A simple seasoning of just salt and pepper allows the natural taste of the scallops to shine.

Serve the pan•seared scallops as a main course with roasted vegetables or a fresh salad. They also make a great appetizer when paired with toothpicks or skewers.

For extra flavor, you can add a sprinkle of lemon zest, chopped parsley, or a drizzle of balsamic glaze over the top of the scallops.

Enjoy this easy, 0 point weight loss recipe for delicious pan•seared scallops!

74. Baked cod with herbs

Ingredients:

• 1 lb cod fillets
• 1 tbsp olive oil
• 2 tbsp chopped fresh parsley
• 1 tbsp chopped fresh dill
• 1 tbsp chopped fresh thyme
• 1 lemon, cut into wedges
• Salt and pepper to taste

Instructions:

1. Preheat your oven to 400°F. Line a baking sheet with parchment paper.

2. Place the cod fillets on the prepared baking sheet. Drizzle the olive oil over the top and use your hands to gently rub it all over the fish.

3. In a small bowl, mix together the chopped parsley, dill, and thyme. Sprinkle this herb mixture evenly over the top of the cod.

4. Season the cod with salt and pepper to taste.

5. Bake the cod for 12•15 minutes, until it flakes easily with a fork and is opaque throughout.

6. Serve the baked cod immediately, with lemon wedges on the side for squeezing over the top.

This baked cod with herbs recipe is a 0 point dish on Weight Watchers. Cod is an excellent source of lean protein that is low in calories and carbs, making it a great choice for weight loss.

The fresh herbs add tons of flavor without any extra calories or points. The lemon wedges provide a bright, acidic contrast that complements the mild, flaky cod.

You can serve the baked cod with roasted vegetables, a side salad, or steamed rice for a complete and nutritious meal. It also makes a great topping for grain bowls or pasta dishes.

For extra flavor, you can also try adding a sprinkle of garlic powder, paprika, or lemon zest to the herb mixture.

75. Tilapia with lemon

Ingredients:

• 4 tilapia fillets (about 1 lb total)
• 2 tbsp olive oil
• 2 tbsp fresh lemon juice
• 1 tsp grated lemon zest
• 2 cloves garlic, minced
• Salt and pepper to taste
• Lemon wedges for serving

Instructions:

1. Preheat your oven to 400°F. Line a baking sheet with parchment paper or foil.

2. In a small bowl, whisk together the olive oil, lemon juice, lemon zest, and minced garlic. Season with a pinch of salt and pepper.

3. Place the tilapia fillets on the prepared baking sheet. Drizzle the lemon•garlic mixture evenly over the top of the fish.

4. Bake for 12•15 minutes, until the tilapia is opaque and flakes easily with a fork.

5. Serve the baked tilapia immediately, with lemon wedges on the side for squeezing over the top.

That's it! This simple tilapia with lemon recipe is a quick and healthy weeknight meal.

Tilapia is a mild, flaky white fish that pairs beautifully with the bright, tangy flavors of lemon. The lemon•garlic sauce keeps the fish moist and infuses it with tons of flavor.

Serve the baked tilapia with roasted vegetables, a fresh salad, or steamed rice for a complete and nutritious meal. The lemon wedges allow you to add an extra pop of citrus to each bite.

This recipe is low in calories and carbs, making it a great option for weight loss or a diabetes•friendly diet. Enjoy this easy and delicious tilapia dish!

76. Lemon garlic shrimp

Ingredients:

• 1 lb large shrimp, peeled and deveined
• 2 tbsp olive oil
• 3 cloves garlic, minced
• 1 tbsp lemon juice
• 1 tsp lemon zest
• 1 tbsp chopped parsley
• Salt and pepper to taste
• Lemon wedges for serving

Instructions:

1. In a large skillet, heat the olive oil over medium•high heat.

2. Add the minced garlic and cook for 1 minute, until fragrant.

3. Add the shrimp to the skillet and cook for 2•3 minutes per side, until the shrimp are pink and opaque.

4. Remove the skillet from the heat and stir in the lemon juice, lemon zest, and chopped parsley. Season with salt and pepper to taste.

5. Serve the lemon garlic shrimp immediately, with lemon wedges on the side.

This lemon garlic shrimp recipe is a quick and easy way to prepare a delicious seafood dish. Shrimp is a lean protein that is low in calories and carbs, making it a great choice for a healthy meal.

The bright, tangy flavors of lemon pair perfectly with the savory garlic. The parsley adds a fresh, herbal note. You can adjust the amount of lemon and garlic to suit your taste preferences.

Serve the lemon garlic shrimp over a bed of zucchini noodles, cauliflower rice, or with a side salad for a complete and nutritious meal. It also makes a great appetizer when served with toothpicks or skewers.

For extra flavor, you can try adding a splash of white wine or a pinch of red pepper flakes to the skillet. This lemon garlic shrimp recipe is sure to become a new favorite!

77. Greek•style grilled chicken

Ingredients:

• 1 lb boneless, skinless chicken breasts
• 2 tbsp olive oil
• 2 tbsp lemon juice
• 1 tbsp dried oregano
• 2 cloves garlic, minced
• 1 tsp salt
• 1/2 tsp black pepper

Instructions:

1. In a shallow baking dish or resealable plastic bag, combine the olive oil, lemon juice, oregano, garlic, salt, and pepper. Add the chicken breasts and turn to coat them evenly in the marinade.

2. Cover the dish or seal the bag and refrigerate for at least 30 minutes, up to 4 hours, to allow the flavors to infuse the chicken.

3. Preheat your grill or grill pan to medium•high heat.

4. Remove the chicken from the marinade and discard any remaining marinade.

5. Grill the chicken for 5•7 minutes per side, until cooked through and no longer pink in the center.

6. Transfer the grilled chicken to a cutting board and let it rest for 5 minutes before slicing or serving.

This Greek•style grilled chicken is a 0 point dish on Weight Watchers. The simple marinade of olive oil, lemon, oregano, and garlic infuses the chicken with tons of Mediterranean flavor without any added calories or points.

Grilling the chicken gives it a nice char and smoky taste. Boneless, skinless chicken breasts are an excellent lean protein source that is low in fat and carbs.

Serve the grilled chicken with roasted vegetables, a Greek salad, or over a bed of leafy greens for a complete and nutritious 0 point meal. You can also slice the chicken and use it in wraps, bowls, or sandwiches.

78. Mediterranean tuna salad

Ingredients:

• 2 (5 oz) cans tuna, drained and flaked
• 1/4 cup diced cucumber
• 1/4 cup diced tomato
• 2 tbsp diced red onion
• 2 tbsp chopped kalamata olives
• 1 tbsp chopped fresh parsley
• 1 tbsp lemon juice
• 1 tbsp red wine vinegar
• 1 tsp olive oil
• Salt and pepper to taste

Instructions:
1. In a medium bowl, combine the flaked tuna, diced cucumber, tomato, red onion, kalamata olives, and chopped parsley.

2. In a small bowl, whisk together the lemon juice, red wine vinegar, and olive oil. Season with a pinch of salt and pepper.

3. Pour the dressing over the tuna salad and gently toss to coat everything evenly.

4. Serve the Mediterranean tuna salad chilled, on a bed of lettuce or stuffed into tomatoes or avocado halves.

This Mediterranean tuna salad is a 0 point dish on Weight Watchers. Tuna is an excellent source of lean protein that is low in calories and carbs. The fresh vegetables, olives, and herbs add tons of flavor without any extra points.

The lemon juice and red wine vinegar dressing provides a bright, tangy contrast to the rich tuna. You can adjust the amount of olive oil to your preference.

This tuna salad makes a great lunch or light dinner option. It's also perfect for meal prepping • just store it in an airtight container in the fridge for up to 3 days.

Serve the Mediterranean tuna salad on its own, or use it as a topping for greens, whole grain crackers, or stuffed into tomatoes or avocado halves. Enjoy this delicious and healthy 0 point weight loss recipe!

79. Waldorf chicken salad (with yogurt dressing)

Ingredients:

- 2 cups cooked, diced chicken breast
- 1 apple, diced
- 1 stalk celery, diced
- 1/4 cup grapes, halved
- 2 tbsp chopped walnuts
- 1/4 cup plain non·fat Greek yogurt
- 1 tbsp lemon juice
- 1 tsp honey
- Salt and pepper to taste

Instructions:

1. In a large bowl, combine the diced chicken, apple, celery, grapes, and walnuts. Toss gently to mix.

2. In a small bowl, whisk together the Greek yogurt, lemon juice, and honey. Season with a pinch of salt and pepper.

3. Pour the yogurt dressing over the chicken salad and toss to coat everything evenly.

4. Serve the Waldorf chicken salad chilled, on a bed of lettuce or in a sandwich thin.

This Waldorf chicken salad is a 0 point dish on Weight Watchers. The Greek yogurt dressing provides creaminess without any added fat or calories. The apples, grapes, celery, and walnuts add crunch, sweetness, and healthy fats.

Chicken is a lean protein that will help keep you feeling full and satisfied. This salad makes a great lunch or light dinner option. You can also serve it as a dip with crunchy veggies.

For extra flavor, you can add a sprinkle of curry powder, dried cranberries, or chopped fresh herbs to the salad. Adjust the amount of dressing to your preference.

Enjoy this delicious and nutritious Waldorf chicken salad for a 0 point weight loss meal!

80. Caprese salad skewers

Ingredients:

• 1 pint cherry or grape tomatoes
• 8 oz fresh mozzarella cheese, cut into 1•inch cubes
• 1/4 cup fresh basil leaves
• 2 tbsp balsamic glaze
• 1 tbsp olive oil
• Salt and pepper to taste

Instructions:

1. Thread the tomatoes, mozzarella cubes, and basil leaves onto small skewers or toothpicks, alternating the ingredients.

2. Arrange the Caprese skewers on a serving platter.

3. Drizzle the balsamic glaze and olive oil over the top of the skewers. Season with a pinch of salt and pepper.

4. Serve the Caprese salad skewers immediately.

These Caprese salad skewers are a fun and easy way to enjoy the classic Italian flavor combination of tomatoes, mozzarella, and basil. They make a great appetizer or side dish.

The bite•sized format is perfect for popping in your mouth. The balsamic glaze and olive oil dressing adds a nice touch of acidity and richness to balance the fresh, creamy flavors.

You can use any type of small tomato, such as cherry, grape, or even mini heirloom varieties. For the mozzarella, look for the small, bite•sized "bocconcini" balls.

These Caprese skewers are a great make•ahead option. Assemble them up to a day in advance and refrigerate until ready to serve. Just drizzle with the balsamic and oil right before serving.

Caprese salad skewers are a simple, elegant, and delicious way to enjoy this classic Italian flavor combination. Enjoy!

81. Stuffed grape leaves (dolmas)

Ingredients:

- 1 (16 oz) jar grape leaves, drained and rinsed
- 1 cup cooked brown rice
- 1/2 cup diced tomatoes
- 1/4 cup chopped onion
- 2 tbsp chopped fresh parsley
- 1 tbsp lemon juice
- 1 tsp olive oil
- Salt and pepper to taste

Instructions:

1. In a medium bowl, mix together the cooked brown rice, diced tomatoes, chopped onion, parsley, lemon juice, and olive oil. Season with salt and pepper.

2. Lay a grape leaf shiny•side down on a flat surface. Place 1•2 tbsp of the rice mixture near the stem end of the leaf.

3. Fold the stem end over the filling, then fold in the sides and roll up the leaf tightly to enclose the filling.

4. Place the stuffed grape leaf seam•side down in a baking dish or serving platter. Repeat with the remaining grape leaves and filling.

5. Serve the stuffed grape leaves (dolmas) chilled or at room temperature.

This recipe for stuffed grape leaves is a 0 point dish on Weight Watchers. The grape leaves are low in calories, while the brown rice, tomatoes, onion, and parsley provide fiber, vitamins, and minerals.

Dolmas make a great appetizer, side dish, or light main course. They are a classic Mediterranean dish that is both flavorful and nutritious.

You can adjust the filling ingredients to your taste, adding things like pine nuts, raisins, or mint. The lemon juice and olive oil provide a bright, tangy dressing for the dolmas.

Serve the stuffed grape leaves with a side of tzatziki sauce or hummus for dipping. They also pair well with pita bread, olives, and feta cheese.

Enjoy this delicious and healthy 0 point weight loss recipe for stuffed grape leaves (dolmas)!

82. Tabbouleh salad

Ingredients:

• 1 cup bulgur wheat
• 1 cup boiling water
• 1 cup finely chopped parsley
• 1/2 cup finely chopped mint
• 1 cup diced tomatoes
• 1/2 cup diced cucumber
• 1/4 cup diced red onion
• 2 tbsp lemon juice
• 2 tbsp olive oil
• 1 tsp ground cumin
• Salt and pepper to taste

Instructions:

1. In a medium bowl, combine the bulgur wheat and boiling water. Cover and let sit for 30 minutes, until the bulgur has absorbed all the water and is tender.

2. Fluff the bulgur with a fork and let it cool slightly.

3. Add the chopped parsley, mint, diced tomatoes, cucumber, and red onion to the bowl with the bulgur.

4. In a small bowl, whisk together the lemon juice, olive oil, and cumin. Season with salt and pepper.

5. Pour the dressing over the tabbouleh salad and toss gently to coat everything evenly.

6. Refrigerate the tabbouleh salad for at least 30 minutes to allow the flavors to meld. Serve chilled or at room temperature.

Tabbouleh is a refreshing Middle Eastern salad made with bulgur wheat, fresh herbs, vegetables, and a bright lemon•based dressing. It makes a great side dish or light main course.

The combination of the nutty bulgur, aromatic herbs, juicy tomatoes, and crunchy cucumbers and onions creates a wonderful balance of textures and flavors. The cumin in the dressing adds an earthy, warm note.

Tabbouleh is a versatile dish that can be customized to your taste. You can add other veggies like bell peppers or radishes, or swap the bulgur for quinoa or couscous. It's also delicious served with pita bread or falafel.

83. Cucumber gazpacho

Ingredients:

- 3 cups diced cucumber
- 1 cup diced tomato
- 1/2 cup diced onion
- 1 garlic clove, minced
- 2 tbsp red wine vinegar
- 1 tbsp olive oil
- 1 tsp salt
- 1/4 tsp black pepper
- 1/4 cup chopped fresh herbs (such as parsley, basil, or cilantro)

Instructions:

1. In a large bowl, combine the diced cucumber, tomato, onion, and garlic.

2. Add the red wine vinegar, olive oil, salt, and pepper. Stir to combine.

3. Stir in the chopped fresh herbs.

4. Cover and refrigerate for at least 30 minutes to allow the flavors to meld.
5. Serve chilled.

This cucumber gazpacho is a refreshing, low•calorie soup that is perfect for weight loss. It's packed with vegetables and has 0 SmartPoints on Weight Watchers. Enjoy!

84. Egg drop soup

Ingredients:

• 4 cups low•sodium chicken or vegetable broth
• 2 eggs, lightly beaten
• 2 tbsp cornstarch
• 1 tbsp soy sauce
• 1 tsp sesame oil
• 1/4 tsp ground white pepper
• 2 green onions, thinly sliced
• Salt to taste

Instructions:

1. In a medium saucepan, bring the broth to a simmer over medium heat.

2. In a small bowl, whisk together the beaten eggs and cornstarch until smooth.

3. Slowly pour the egg mixture into the simmering broth in a circular motion, while gently stirring the broth with a fork or chopsticks. This will create delicate strands of egg.

4. Stir in the soy sauce, sesame oil, and white pepper. Taste and adjust seasoning with salt as needed.

5. Remove the soup from heat and ladle into bowls. Top with the sliced green onions.

6. Serve the egg drop soup hot.

This classic Chinese egg drop soup is a simple, comforting dish that's easy to make at home. The key is to slowly drizzle the egg mixture into the hot broth to create those delicate egg ribbons.

The soy sauce, sesame oil, and white pepper provide authentic Asian flavors, while the green onions add a fresh, crunchy garnish.

Egg drop soup is a great low•calorie, low•carb option that's perfect for a light meal or starter. It's also naturally gluten•free.

You can customize the soup by adding other ingredients like mushrooms, spinach, or shredded chicken. Adjust the seasoning to your taste.

85. Vietnamese pho (with lean protein)

Ingredients:

• 8 cups low•sodium beef or chicken broth
• 2 whole star anise
• 2 cinnamon sticks
• 1 tablespoon whole coriander seeds
• 1 tablespoon whole fennel seeds
• 1 tablespoon whole cloves
• 1 tablespoon whole black peppercorns
• 1 onion, halved
• 3 garlic cloves, peeled
• 1 (3•inch) piece fresh ginger, peeled and sliced
• 8 oz lean beef sirloin or chicken breast, thinly sliced
• 8 oz whole wheat or brown rice noodles
• 2 cups bean sprouts
• 1 cup fresh cilantro leaves
• 1 cup fresh basil leaves
• 2 green onions, sliced
• 2 lime wedges

Instructions:

1. In a large pot, combine the broth, star anise, cinnamon sticks, coriander seeds, fennel seeds, cloves, peppercorns, onion, garlic, and ginger. Bring to a boil, then reduce heat and simmer for 30 minutes.

2. Strain the broth through a fine mesh sieve, discarding the solids. Return the broth to the pot and bring back to a simmer.

3. Add the sliced beef or chicken and cook for 2•3 minutes until cooked through.

4. Meanwhile, cook the noodles according to package instructions. Drain and rinse with cold water.

5. To serve, divide the noodles and broth between bowls. Top with bean sprouts, cilantro, basil, and green onions. Serve with lime wedges.

This pho is a hearty, flavorful dish that is 0 SmartPoints on Weight Watchers. The lean protein and veggie•packed broth make it a great option for weight loss.

86. Tom yum soup (broth•based)

Ingredients:

• 4 cups low•sodium chicken or vegetable broth
• 2 lemongrass stalks, bruised
• 3 kaffir lime leaves
• 2 slices fresh galangal or ginger
• 2 Thai chilies, sliced (or 1/2 tsp red pepper flakes)
• 2 tbsp fish sauce
• 1 tbsp lime juice
• 1 tsp brown sugar
• 8 oz shrimp, peeled and deveined
• 1 cup sliced mushrooms
• 2 green onions, sliced
• 1/4 cup fresh cilantro leaves

Instructions:

1. In a large pot, combine the broth, lemongrass, lime leaves, galangal/ginger, and chilies. Bring to a boil over high heat.

2. Reduce heat to medium•low and simmer for 10 minutes to allow the flavors to infuse the broth.

3. Stir in the fish sauce, lime juice, and brown sugar. Taste and adjust seasoning as needed.

4. Add the shrimp and mushrooms and cook for 2•3 minutes until the shrimp are opaque.

5. Remove from heat and stir in the green onions and cilantro.

6. Ladle the soup into bowls and serve hot.

This Tom Yum soup is a flavorful, broth•based soup that is 0 SmartPoints on Weight Watchers. The lemongrass, lime, and chili give it a signature Thai flavor. Enjoy this light and healthy soup!

87. Cold sesame noodles (with low•sodium soy sauce)

Ingredients:

• 8 oz whole wheat spaghetti or linguine, cooked according to package instructions and chilled
• 2 tbsp low•sodium soy sauce
• 2 tbsp rice vinegar
• 1 tbsp sesame oil
• 1 tbsp natural peanut butter
• 1 tsp honey
• 1 garlic clove, minced
• 1/4 tsp crushed red pepper flakes (optional)
• 2 cups shredded cabbage or coleslaw mix
• 2 green onions, sliced
• 2 tbsp chopped cilantro (optional)
• 2 tbsp toasted sesame seeds

Instructions:

1. In a medium bowl, whisk together the low•sodium soy sauce, rice vinegar, sesame oil, peanut butter, honey, garlic, and red pepper flakes (if using).

2. Add the cooked and chilled noodles, cabbage/coleslaw, green onions, and cilantro (if using). Toss to coat everything evenly in the sauce.

3. Top with toasted sesame seeds before serving.

This cold sesame noodle dish is refreshing and flavorful. The low•sodium soy sauce keeps the sodium content in check. Enjoy this as a light main dish or side.

88. Asian slaw (with ginger dressing)

Ingredients:

• 2 cups shredded green cabbage
• 2 cups shredded red cabbage
• 1 cup shredded carrots
• 1/2 cup thinly sliced red onion
• 1/4 cup chopped fresh cilantro
• 2 tbsp toasted sesame seeds

Ginger Dressing:
• 2 tbsp rice vinegar
• 1 tbsp low•sodium soy sauce
• 1 tbsp sesame oil
• 1 tbsp honey
• 1 tbsp freshly grated ginger
• 1 garlic clove, minced
• 1/4 tsp crushed red pepper flakes (optional)
• Salt and pepper to taste

Instructions:

1. In a large bowl, combine the shredded green cabbage, red cabbage, carrots, red onion, cilantro, and sesame seeds. Toss to mix.

2. In a small bowl, whisk together all the dressing ingredients • rice vinegar, soy sauce, sesame oil, honey, grated ginger, garlic, and red pepper flakes (if using). Season with salt and pepper.

3. Pour the ginger dressing over the slaw and toss to coat everything evenly.

4. Cover and refrigerate for at least 30 minutes to allow the flavors to meld.

5. Serve chilled or at room temperature.

This Asian slaw makes a great side dish or topping for grilled proteins. The ginger dressing adds a nice zing. It's a refreshing, low•calorie option that's perfect for weight loss.

89. Grilled pineapple salsa

Ingredients:

• 1 fresh pineapple, cut into 1•inch thick slices
• 1 jalapeño, seeded and finely chopped
• 1/2 red onion, finely chopped
• 1/4 cup chopped cilantro
• 2 tbsp lime juice
• Salt and pepper to taste

Instructions:

1. Preheat your grill or grill pan to medium•high heat.

2. Grill the pineapple slices for 2•3 minutes per side, until lightly charred and softened. Allow to cool slightly, then dice the grilled pineapple.

3. In a medium bowl, combine the diced grilled pineapple, chopped jalapeño, red onion, cilantro, and lime juice. Toss gently to mix.

4. Season the pineapple salsa with salt and pepper to taste.

5. Serve the grilled pineapple salsa immediately, or refrigerate until ready to use.

This grilled pineapple salsa is a 0 point dish on Weight Watchers. Pineapple is naturally sweet and low in calories, while the jalapeño, onion, and lime juice add a refreshing, zesty kick.

The grilling adds a nice smoky depth of flavor to the pineapple. You can adjust the amount of jalapeño to control the spice level.

Serve the grilled pineapple salsa as a topping for grilled fish or chicken, or enjoy it with baked tortilla chips for a healthy snack. It also makes a great addition to tacos, burrito bowls, or salads.

For extra flavor, you can try adding a pinch of cumin, chili powder, or chopped fresh herbs to the salsa.

Enjoy this delicious and nutritious 0 point weight loss recipe for grilled pineapple salsa!

90. Marinated olives

Ingredients:

• 1 cup mixed olives (such as Kalamata, green, and/or black olives), pitted and halved
• 2 tbsp olive oil
• 1 tbsp red wine vinegar
• 1 garlic clove, minced
• 1 tsp dried oregano
• 1/4 tsp red pepper flakes (optional)
• 1 bay leaf
• Zest of 1 lemon
• Salt and pepper to taste

Instructions:

1. In a medium bowl, combine the halved olives, olive oil, red wine vinegar, garlic, oregano, red pepper flakes (if using), bay leaf, and lemon zest. Stir to coat the olives evenly.

2. Season with salt and pepper to taste.

3. Cover the bowl and refrigerate for at least 30 minutes, or up to 1 week, to allow the flavors to meld.

4. When ready to serve, remove the bay leaf. Taste and adjust seasoning if needed.

5. Serve the marinated olives at room temperature or chilled, as an appetizer or side dish.

These marinated olives make a great healthy snack or appetizer. The olive oil, vinegar, herbs, and spices infuse the olives with lots of flavor. They are 0 SmartPoints on Weight Watchers, so they are a perfect option for weight loss. Enjoy!

91. Roasted beet salad

Ingredients:

- 3 medium beets, peeled and cut into 1·inch cubes
- 1 tbsp olive oil
- 1/4 tsp salt
- 1/8 tsp black pepper
- 4 cups mixed greens (such as spinach, arugula, or kale)
- 2 tbsp crumbled feta cheese (optional)
- 2 tbsp chopped walnuts (optional)
- 2 tbsp balsamic vinegar

Instructions:

1. Preheat your oven to 400°F (200°C). Line a baking sheet with parchment paper.

2. In a medium bowl, toss the cubed beets with the olive oil, salt, and pepper until evenly coated.

3. Spread the seasoned beets in a single layer on the prepared baking sheet.

4. Roast the beets in the preheated oven for 20·25 minutes, stirring halfway, until they are tender and lightly caramelized.

5. Remove the roasted beets from the oven and let them cool slightly.

6. In a large salad bowl, combine the mixed greens, roasted beets, feta cheese (if using), and walnuts (if using).

7. Drizzle the balsamic vinegar over the salad and toss gently to coat.

8. Serve the roasted beet salad immediately.

This roasted beet salad is a delicious and nutritious 0 SmartPoint dish on the Weight Watchers program. The sweet, earthy beets pair perfectly with the tangy balsamic vinegar and optional feta and walnuts. Enjoy this flavorful and satisfying salad!

92. Roasted fennel

Ingredients:

• 2 medium fennel bulbs, trimmed and cut into 1/2•inch thick slices
• 1 tbsp olive oil
• 1/2 tsp salt
• 1/4 tsp black pepper
• 1 tbsp chopped fresh parsley (optional)

Instructions:

1. Preheat your oven to 400°F (200°C).

2. Arrange the fennel slices in a single layer on a baking sheet lined with parchment paper or a silicone baking mat.

3. Drizzle the fennel with the olive oil and sprinkle with salt and black pepper. Toss to coat the fennel evenly.

4. Roast the fennel in the preheated oven for 20•25 minutes, flipping halfway, until it's tender and lightly browned.

5. Remove the roasted fennel from the oven and transfer it to a serving dish.

6. If desired, sprinkle the roasted fennel with the chopped fresh parsley.

7. Serve the roasted fennel warm or at room temperature.

This roasted fennel dish is a simple and delicious way to enjoy this vegetable. It's 0 SmartPoints on the Weight Watchers program, making it a great option for weight loss. The fennel becomes sweet and caramelized in the oven, and the parsley adds a fresh, herbal note.

93. Roasted acorn squash

Ingredients:

• 1 acorn squash, halved and seeded
• Nonstick cooking spray
• Salt and pepper to taste

Instructions:

1. Preheat your oven to 400°F. Line a baking sheet with parchment paper.

2. Cut the acorn squash in half lengthwise and scoop out the seeds. Place the squash halves cut·side up on the prepared baking sheet.

3. Lightly spray the squash halves with nonstick cooking spray and season with salt and pepper.

4. Roast the acorn squash for 30·40 minutes, until fork·tender.

5. Remove the roasted squash from the oven and let it cool slightly. Serve warm.

This roasted acorn squash recipe is a 0 point dish on Weight Watchers. Acorn squash is a nutrient·dense winter squash that is low in calories and carbs, making it an excellent choice for weight loss.

The simple preparation of just spraying with nonstick cooking spray and seasoning with salt and pepper allows the natural sweetness and creamy texture of the squash to shine.

You can enjoy the roasted acorn squash halves as a side dish, or scoop out the flesh and mash it for a comforting, low·calorie side. It also makes a great base for soups, stews, or grain bowls.

For extra flavor, you can try drizzling the roasted squash with a bit of maple syrup, cinnamon, or a sprinkle of parmesan cheese. But the squash is delicious on its own as well.

This 0 point weight loss recipe for roasted acorn squash is an easy and versatile way to enjoy this nutritious winter vegetable. Enjoy!

94. Roasted butternut squash

Ingredients:

• 1 medium butternut squash, peeled, seeded, and cut into 1•inch cubes (about 4 cups)
• 1 tbsp olive oil
• 1/2 tsp salt
• 1/4 tsp black pepper
• 1 tbsp chopped fresh thyme (optional)

Instructions:

1. Preheat your oven to 400°F (200°C). Line a baking sheet with parchment paper or a silicone baking mat.

2. In a large bowl, toss the cubed butternut squash with the olive oil, salt, and black pepper until the squash is evenly coated.

3. Spread the seasoned butternut squash in a single layer on the prepared baking sheet.

4. Roast the squash in the preheated oven for 25•30 minutes, flipping halfway, until it is tender and lightly browned.

5. Remove the roasted butternut squash from the oven and transfer it to a serving dish.

6. If desired, sprinkle the roasted squash with the chopped fresh thyme.

7. Serve the roasted butternut squash warm.

This roasted butternut squash is a delicious and nutritious side dish that is 0 SmartPoints on the Weight Watchers program. The natural sweetness of the squash is enhanced by the roasting process, making it a great option for weight loss. Enjoy this simple and flavorful dish!

95. Roasted turnips

Ingredients:

- 1 lb turnips, peeled and cut into 1·inch cubes
- 1 tbsp olive oil
- 1/2 tsp salt
- 1/4 tsp black pepper
- 1 tbsp chopped fresh parsley (optional)

Instructions:

1. Preheat your oven to 400°F (200°C). Line a baking sheet with parchment paper or a silicone baking mat.

2. In a large bowl, toss the cubed turnips with the olive oil, salt, and black pepper until they are evenly coated.

3. Spread the seasoned turnips in a single layer on the prepared baking sheet.

4. Roast the turnips in the preheated oven for 20·25 minutes, flipping halfway, until they are tender and lightly browned.

5. Remove the roasted turnips from the oven and transfer them to a serving dish.

6. If desired, sprinkle the roasted turnips with the chopped fresh parsley.

7. Serve the roasted turnips warm.

These roasted turnips are a delicious and healthy side dish that is 0 SmartPoints on the Weight Watchers program. The turnips become tender and caramelized in the oven, with a slightly sweet and earthy flavor. They make a great alternative to potatoes for a low·calorie option.

96. Roasted parsnips

Ingredients:

• 1 lb parsnips, peeled and cut into 1•inch pieces
• 1 tbsp olive oil
• 1/2 tsp salt
• 1/4 tsp black pepper
• 1 tbsp chopped fresh parsley (optional)

Instructions:

1. Preheat your oven to 400°F (200°C). Line a baking sheet with parchment paper or a silicone baking mat.

2. In a large bowl, toss the parsnip pieces with the olive oil, salt, and black pepper until they are evenly coated.

3. Spread the seasoned parsnips in a single layer on the prepared baking sheet.

4. Roast the parsnips in the preheated oven for 20•25 minutes, flipping halfway, until they are tender and lightly browned.

5. Remove the roasted parsnips from the oven and transfer them to a serving dish.

6. If desired, sprinkle the roasted parsnips with the chopped fresh parsley.

7. Serve the roasted parsnips warm.

These roasted parsnips are a delicious and healthy side dish that is 0 SmartPoints on the Weight Watchers program. The natural sweetness of the parsnips is enhanced by the roasting process, making them a great option for weight loss. Enjoy!

97. Miso soup

Ingredients:

- 4 cups low•sodium vegetable or chicken broth
- 2 tbsp white or yellow miso paste
- 1 cup cubed firm tofu
- 1 cup sliced mushrooms
- 1 cup chopped spinach or kale
- 2 green onions, sliced
- 1 tsp grated fresh ginger (optional)

Instructions:

1. In a medium saucepan, bring the broth to a gentle simmer over medium heat.

2. In a small bowl, whisk together the miso paste with a few tablespoons of the hot broth until smooth.

3. Carefully pour the miso mixture back into the saucepan with the broth, whisking to incorporate.

4. Add the cubed tofu, mushrooms, and greens (spinach or kale) to the broth. Simmer for 2•3 minutes until the greens are wilted.

5. Remove from heat and stir in the sliced green onions.

6. If desired, stir in the grated fresh ginger.

7. Ladle the miso soup into bowls and serve hot.

This miso soup is a simple, flavorful, and nourishing dish that is 0 SmartPoints on Weight Watchers. The miso paste provides umami flavor, while the tofu, mushrooms, and greens make it a satisfying and healthy meal. Enjoy this comforting soup!

98. Cauliflower steaks

Ingredients:

• 1 large head of cauliflower, cut into 1•inch thick slices (cauliflower "steaks")
• 2 tbsp olive oil
• 1 tsp garlic powder
• 1 tsp paprika
• 1/2 tsp salt
• 1/4 tsp black pepper

Instructions:

1. Preheat your oven to 400°F (200°C). Line a baking sheet with parchment paper or a silicone baking mat.

2. Carefully slice the cauliflower head from top to bottom, creating 1•inch thick "steaks". Try to get 4•6 steaks from the head.

3. Arrange the cauliflower steaks in a single layer on the prepared baking sheet.

4. In a small bowl, mix together the olive oil, garlic powder, paprika, salt, and black pepper.

5. Brush or drizzle the seasoned oil mixture over the top of the cauliflower steaks, making sure to coat them evenly on both sides.

6. Roast the cauliflower steaks in the preheated oven for 20•25 minutes, flipping halfway, until they are tender and lightly browned on the edges.

7. Serve the roasted cauliflower steaks warm, garnished with fresh herbs if desired.

These cauliflower steaks are a delicious and healthy alternative to traditional meat•based steaks. They are 0 SmartPoints on the Weight Watchers program, making them a great option for weight loss. Enjoy them as a main dish or side.

99. Chickpea salad

Ingredients:

- 1 (15 oz) can chickpeas, drained and rinsed
- 1/2 cup diced cucumber
- 1/2 cup diced tomatoes
- 1/4 cup diced red onion
- 2 tbsp chopped fresh parsley
- 1 tbsp lemon juice
- 1 tsp Dijon mustard
- 1 garlic clove, minced
- 1/4 tsp salt
- 1/8 tsp black pepper

Instructions:

1. In a medium bowl, combine the drained and rinsed chickpeas, diced cucumber, tomatoes, red onion, and chopped parsley.

2. In a small bowl, whisk together the lemon juice, Dijon mustard, minced garlic, salt, and black pepper to make the dressing.

3. Pour the dressing over the chickpea salad and toss gently to coat the ingredients evenly.

4. Cover and refrigerate the chickpea salad for at least 30 minutes to allow the flavors to meld.

5. Serve the chilled chickpea salad as a side dish or light main course.

This chickpea salad is a delicious and nutritious 0 SmartPoint dish on the Weight Watchers program. The chickpeas provide protein and fiber, while the fresh vegetables and tangy dressing add lots of flavor. It's a great option for a healthy, filling meal or snack.

100. Eggplant caponata

Ingredients:

- 1 medium eggplant, diced
- 1 tbsp olive oil
- 1 onion, diced
- 2 cloves garlic, minced
- 1 (14 oz) can diced tomatoes
- 2 tbsp red wine vinegar
- 1 tbsp capers, rinsed and chopped
- 2 tbsp chopped fresh basil
- Salt and pepper to taste

Instructions:

1. In a large skillet, heat the olive oil over medium heat. Add the diced eggplant and cook for 5•7 minutes, stirring occasionally, until softened.

2. Add the diced onion and minced garlic to the skillet. Cook for 2•3 minutes more, until the onion is translucent.

3. Pour in the can of diced tomatoes along with their juices. Stir in the red wine vinegar and chopped capers.

4. Reduce the heat to low and let the caponata simmer for 15•20 minutes, stirring occasionally, until the flavors have melded and the mixture has thickened.

5. Remove from heat and stir in the chopped fresh basil. Season with salt and pepper to taste.

6. Serve the eggplant caponata warm or at room temperature. It can be enjoyed on its own, with crusty bread, or as a topping for grilled fish or chicken.

This eggplant caponata is a 0 point dish on Weight Watchers. Eggplant is the star ingredient, providing fiber, vitamins, and a meaty texture. The tomatoes, vinegar, and herbs add tons of flavor without any extra calories or points.

Caponata is a classic Sicilian dish that makes a great appetizer, side, or light main course. The sweet, sour, and savory flavors pair beautifully together.

For extra crunch, you can add toasted pine nuts or chopped walnuts to the caponata. Adjust the amount of vinegar to your taste preference.

101. Spinach and feta stuffed mushrooms

Ingredients:

- 12 large mushrooms, stems removed and finely chopped
- 1 tsp olive oil
- 1/4 cup finely chopped onion
- 2 garlic cloves, minced
- 1 cup fresh spinach, chopped
- 2 oz crumbled feta cheese
- 2 tbsp grated Parmesan cheese
- 1/4 tsp dried oregano
- Salt and pepper to taste

Instructions:

1. Preheat your oven to 375°F (190°C). Line a baking sheet with parchment paper.

2. Gently clean the mushroom caps with a damp paper towel. Carefully remove the stems and finely chop them.

3. In a skillet, heat the olive oil over medium heat. Add the chopped mushroom stems, onion, and garlic. Sauté for 2•3 minutes until softened.

4. Add the chopped spinach to the skillet and cook for 1•2 minutes until wilted. Remove from heat and let cool slightly.

5. In a small bowl, mix the sautéed mushroom stem mixture with the crumbled feta, Parmesan, and dried oregano. Season with salt and pepper to taste.

6. Spoon the spinach and feta filling into the mushroom caps, dividing it evenly.

7. Arrange the stuffed mushrooms on the prepared baking sheet.

8. Bake for 12•15 minutes, until the mushrooms are tender and the filling is hot.

9. Serve the spinach and feta stuffed mushrooms warm.

These stuffed mushrooms make a delicious and healthy appetizer or side dish. Enjoy!

102. Shrimp stir•fry (with vegetables)

Ingredients:

• 1 lb raw shrimp, peeled and deveined
• 2 cups mixed vegetables (such as broccoli florets, sliced bell peppers, snow peas, and sliced mushrooms)
• 1 tbsp low•sodium soy sauce
• 1 tbsp rice vinegar
• 1 tsp sesame oil
• 1 garlic clove, minced
• 1 tsp grated fresh ginger
• 1/4 tsp red pepper flakes (optional)
• Salt and pepper to taste
• Chopped green onions and sesame seeds for garnish (optional)

Instructions:

1. In a large non•stick skillet or wok, stir•fry the mixed vegetables over high heat for 3•4 minutes until crisp•tender. Transfer to a plate.

2. In the same skillet, add the shrimp and stir•fry for 2•3 minutes until the shrimp start to turn pink.

3. Add the soy sauce, rice vinegar, sesame oil, garlic, ginger, and red pepper flakes (if using). Stir•fry for 1•2 minutes until the shrimp are cooked through.

4. Return the cooked vegetables to the skillet and toss everything together until heated through.

5. Season with salt and pepper to taste.

6. Serve the shrimp stir•fry hot, garnished with chopped green onions and sesame seeds if desired.

This shrimp stir•fry is a delicious and healthy 0 SmartPoint dish on Weight Watchers. The lean protein from the shrimp and the fiber•rich vegetables make it a satisfying meal option for weight loss.

103. Chicken lettuce wraps

Ingredients:

- 1 lb ground chicken or finely chopped chicken breast
- 1 tbsp sesame oil
- 2 garlic cloves, minced
- 1 tbsp grated fresh ginger
- 2 tbsp low•sodium soy sauce
- 1 tbsp rice vinegar
- 1 tsp honey
- 1/4 tsp red pepper flakes (optional)
- 1 cup shredded carrots
- 1 cup thinly sliced mushrooms
- 1/2 cup diced water chestnuts
- 1/4 cup chopped green onions
- 12•16 large lettuce leaves (such as romaine, bibb, or butter lettuce)

Instructions:

1. In a large skillet or wok, cook the ground chicken over medium•high heat, breaking it up with a wooden spoon, until no longer pink, about 5•7 minutes. Drain any excess liquid.

2. Add the sesame oil, garlic, and ginger to the skillet. Cook for 1 minute, stirring constantly, until fragrant.

3. Stir in the soy sauce, rice vinegar, honey, and red pepper flakes (if using). Bring the mixture to a simmer and cook for 2•3 minutes.

4. Add the shredded carrots, sliced mushrooms, water chestnuts, and green onions. Toss to combine and cook for 2•3 minutes more.

5. To serve, spoon the chicken mixture into the lettuce leaves. Wrap the lettuce around the filling and enjoy.

These chicken lettuce wraps are a delicious and healthy meal option. The lean protein from the chicken, crunchy vegetables, and fresh lettuce leaves make them a great choice for weight loss. Enjoy!

104. Greek yogurt with berries

Ingredients:

• 1 cup plain non•fat Greek yogurt
• 1 cup mixed fresh berries (such as blueberries, raspberries, blackberries)
• 1 tsp honey (optional)

Instructions:

1. Spoon the Greek yogurt into a serving bowl or parfait glass.

2. Top the yogurt with the mixed fresh berries.

3. If desired, drizzle a teaspoon of honey over the top.

That's it! This Greek yogurt with berries is a simple, healthy, and delicious 0 point weight loss snack or breakfast.

Greek yogurt is an excellent source of protein, calcium, and probiotics. Pairing it with fresh, antioxidant•rich berries makes for a nutritious and satisfying treat.

The honey is optional, as the natural sweetness of the berries can be enough. But a small drizzle can add a nice touch of sweetness if desired.

You can use any combination of fresh berries you like • strawberries, blueberries, raspberries, and blackberries all work well. Frozen berries can also be used if fresh are not available.

This Greek yogurt with berries is a versatile dish that can be enjoyed on its own or as part of a larger meal. It's perfect for breakfast, a snack, or even a light dessert.

Enjoy this easy, 0 point weight loss recipe for a delicious and healthy Greek yogurt with berries!

105. Avocado salad

Ingredients:

- 2 ripe avocados, diced
- 1 cup cherry tomatoes, halved
- 1/4 cup diced red onion
- 2 tbsp chopped fresh cilantro
- 1 tbsp lime juice
- 1 tsp olive oil
- 1/4 tsp salt
- 1/8 tsp black pepper

Instructions:

1. In a medium bowl, gently toss together the diced avocados, cherry tomatoes, red onion, and chopped cilantro.

2. Drizzle the lime juice and olive oil over the salad and season with salt and black pepper.

3. Toss the salad gently to coat the ingredients evenly with the dressing.

4. Serve the avocado salad immediately or refrigerate until ready to serve.

This simple avocado salad is a refreshing and nutritious dish. The creamy avocado, juicy tomatoes, and tangy lime dressing make a delicious flavor combination.

This salad is a great source of healthy fats, vitamins, and antioxidants. It's a perfect side dish or light main course that's also 0 SmartPoints on the Weight Watchers program, making it a great option for weight loss.

You can customize the salad by adding other veggies like cucumber, bell peppers, or leafy greens. Enjoy this easy and flavorful avocado salad!

106. Cabbage salad with apple cider vinaigrette

Ingredients:

• 4 cups shredded green cabbage
• 2 cups shredded red cabbage
• 1 cup shredded carrots
• 1/2 cup thinly sliced red onion
• 2 tbsp chopped fresh parsley

Vinaigrette Ingredients:
• 2 tbsp apple cider vinegar
• 1 tbsp Dijon mustard
• 1 tbsp honey
• 1 tbsp olive oil
• 1/4 tsp salt
• 1/8 tsp black pepper

Instructions:

1. In a large bowl, combine the shredded green cabbage, red cabbage, carrots, red onion, and parsley. Toss to mix.

2. In a small bowl, whisk together the apple cider vinegar, Dijon mustard, honey, olive oil, salt, and black pepper to make the vinaigrette.

3. Pour the vinaigrette over the cabbage salad and toss to coat the vegetables evenly.

4. Cover and refrigerate the cabbage salad for at least 30 minutes to allow the flavors to meld.

5. Serve the chilled cabbage salad as a side dish.

This cabbage salad with apple cider vinaigrette is a refreshing and flavorful 0 point dish on the Weight Watchers program. The crunchy cabbage and carrots paired with the tangy vinaigrette make it a perfect light and healthy side. It's a great option for summer meals or as part of a weight loss•friendly meal plan.

107. Lentil tabbouleh

Ingredients:

- 1 cup cooked brown or green lentils, cooled
- 1 cup chopped fresh parsley
- 1/2 cup chopped fresh mint
- 1 cup diced tomatoes
- 1/2 cup diced cucumber
- 1/4 cup diced red onion
- 2 tbsp lemon juice
- 1 tbsp olive oil
- 1 garlic clove, minced
- 1/4 tsp salt
- 1/8 tsp black pepper

Instructions:

1. In a large bowl, combine the cooked and cooled lentils, chopped parsley, mint, diced tomatoes, cucumber, and red onion.

2. In a small bowl, whisk together the lemon juice, olive oil, minced garlic, salt, and black pepper to make the dressing.

3. Pour the dressing over the lentil and vegetable mixture and toss gently to coat everything evenly.

4. Cover and refrigerate the lentil tabbouleh for at least 30 minutes to allow the flavors to meld.

5. Serve the chilled lentil tabbouleh as a side dish or light main course.

This lentil tabbouleh is a delicious and nutritious salad that is 0 SmartPoints on the Weight Watchers program. The lentils provide plant•based protein and fiber, while the fresh herbs, vegetables, and tangy dressing make it a flavorful and refreshing dish. It's a great option for a healthy, filling meal or side.

108. Cucumber salad with dill

Ingredients:

• 2 medium cucumbers, thinly sliced
• 1/2 red onion, thinly sliced
• 2 tbsp white wine vinegar
• 1 tbsp fresh dill, chopped
• 1 tsp Dijon mustard
• 1 tsp honey
• 1/4 tsp salt
• 1/8 tsp black pepper

Instructions:

1. In a large bowl, combine the thinly sliced cucumbers and red onion.

2. In a small bowl, whisk together the white wine vinegar, chopped dill, Dijon mustard, honey, salt, and black pepper.

3. Pour the dressing over the cucumber and onion mixture and toss gently to coat.

4. Cover and refrigerate the cucumber salad for at least 30 minutes, or up to 2 hours, to allow the flavors to meld.

5. Serve the chilled cucumber salad as a side dish.

This cucumber salad with dill is a refreshing and flavorful 0 point dish on the Weight Watchers program. The tangy vinegar dressing, fresh dill, and crunchy cucumbers make it a perfect light and healthy side. It's a great option for summer meals or as part of a weight loss•friendly meal plan.

109. Chia seed pudding (with almond milk)

Ingredients:

• 2 cups unsweetened almond milk
• 1/4 cup chia seeds
• 1 tsp vanilla extract
• 1/2 tsp ground cinnamon (optional)
• Fresh berries or sliced fruit for topping (optional)

Instructions:

1. In a medium bowl, whisk together the almond milk, chia seeds, vanilla extract, and cinnamon (if using) until well combined.

2. Cover the bowl and refrigerate for at least 4 hours, or overnight, stirring occasionally, until the chia seeds have thickened the mixture into a pudding•like consistency.

3. Divide the chia seed pudding into individual serving bowls or containers.

4. Top the chia pudding with your choice of fresh berries or sliced fruit, if desired.

5. Serve chilled.

This chia seed pudding is a delicious and nutritious 0 SmartPoint breakfast or snack on the Weight Watchers program. The chia seeds provide fiber, protein, and healthy omega•3s, while the unsweetened almond milk keeps it low in calories and points. Feel free to adjust the amount of chia seeds or add your favorite toppings to suit your taste preferences.

110. Apple slices with cinnamon

Ingredients:

• 2 medium apples, cored and sliced
• 1/2 tsp ground cinnamon

Instructions:

1. Wash and core the apples, then slice them into thin wedges or rounds.

2. Arrange the apple slices on a plate or platter.

3. Sprinkle the ground cinnamon evenly over the apple slices.

4. Serve immediately or refrigerate until ready to enjoy.

That's it! This is a super easy and healthy 0 SmartPoint snack or dessert on the Weight Watchers program.

The natural sweetness of the apples paired with the warm cinnamon flavor makes this a delicious and satisfying treat. It's a great option when you're craving something sweet but want to keep it low in calories and points.

You can enjoy the apple slices on their own or try dipping them in a bit of low•fat Greek yogurt for added protein and creaminess. This simple snack is perfect for weight loss or as a healthy alternative to higher calorie desserts.

*Congratulations on reaching the conclusion of the **"Zero Point Weight Loss Cookbook: Satisfying and Nutritious Meals for Every Occasion."** We hope that this journey through over 110 delicious, zero point recipes has been as enjoyable and enlightening for you as it has been for us to compile.*

By now, you've experienced firsthand how easy and rewarding it can be to create meals that are both healthy and satisfying. The recipes in this cookbook are designed not just to help you lose weight, but to foster a lasting, positive relationship with food. Each dish was crafted to be flavorful and nourishing, demonstrating that weight loss doesn't have to mean compromising on taste or pleasure.

Throughout this cookbook, we've aimed to provide you with a diverse range of meals that fit seamlessly into your everyday life, whether you're cooking for yourself, your family, or entertaining guests. We've shown that eating well can be simple, delicious, and joyful, regardless of the occasion.

As you continue on your journey towards better health, we encourage you to revisit these recipes often and experiment with new ones. Use the knowledge and skills you've gained to make mindful choices and to explore the endless possibilities that come with a zero point approach to eating. Remember, this is more than just a diet; it's a sustainable way to enjoy food while achieving your wellness goals.

We hope that this cookbook has inspired you to take control of your health in a way that feels both manageable and fulfilling. The path to weight loss and wellness is a personal one, and we are honored to have been a part of your journey.

Thank you for allowing us to be a part of your kitchen and your life. We wish you continued success and satisfaction as you move forward, creating meals that nourish both body and soul. Here's to a healthier, happier you—one zero point meal at a time.

Bon appétit!